MENTAL HEALTH
A Pocket Guide **4e**

MENTAL HEALTH
A Pocket Guide 4e

Deb O'Kane

ELSEVIER

ELSEVIER

Elsevier Australia. ACN 001 002 357
(a division of Reed International Books Australia Pty Ltd)
Tower 1, 475 Victoria Avenue, Chatswood, NSW 2067

ISBN: 978-0-7295-4403-0

Notice

National Library of Australia Cataloguing-in-Publication Data

A catalogue record for this book is available from the National Library of Australia

---

Senior Content Strategist: Libby Houston
Content Project Manager: Shubham Dixit
Edited by Jo Crichton
Proofread by Melissa Faulkner
Cover and design by Lisa Petroff
Index by Innodata Indexing
Typeset by GW Tech
Printed in India by Multivista Global Pvt. Ltd

Last digit is the print number: 9 8 7 6 5 4 3 2 1

FOREWORD

This pocket guide is the most useful resource I have seen for anyone working in or entering the field of mental health practice. The information covered is so accessible that I would recommend it to anyone who wants to understand what holistic, modern, mental healthcare should look like. This includes the people in contact with mental health services, their families, and people who work across the health and social care system more broadly.

The chapters capture the fundamental essence of all that is important to delivering effective, ethical and humane care for people with mental illness. They take the reader directly and succinctly to key areas of the most current international focus, and to evidence for the practices that guide mental healthcare delivery and how holistic care should be delivered.

Importantly, the contents of this pocket guide do not see the person in isolation from their friends, family and community; the many important foundations for 'lived experience' that contribute to mental health across the lifespan are discussed. These provide the essential holistic context in which clinical care aspects are also discussed. Also important is the clarity in describing the essential attitudes and beliefs that underpin practice as part of working within a healthcare delivery culture that genuinely places the person's needs and preferences at its core.

I commend this pocket guide to you.

Professor Sharon Lawn
Former SA Mental Health Commissioner,
Researcher and Lived Experience Advocate

PREFACE

Approximately 792 million people worldwide have a mental health problem, and over 75% of these problems occur before the age of 25. For these reasons, mental health and illness awareness are fundamental to all those working in health and health-related areas. This handy, readable text is intended to provide easy access to immediate advice for a range of health professionals and workers, including general nurses, general practitioners, paramedics, police, mental health workers, drug and alcohol workers and allied health professionals who encounter people with mental health problems in their daily work. This text will also be useful for mental health support workers and those in consumer care roles. The core elements of engaging and working with people with mental health problems are distilled into practical skills and approaches that can be applied to a range of care settings.

This fourth edition has been comprehensively prepared to provide the latest evidence about mental healthcare and includes new chapters and more detail in the areas of trauma-informed care and loss in the face of natural disasters.

At the core of mental health practice is a focus on social inclusion, person-centred care and recovery, cultural understanding and respect for and promotion of consumer rights. Accordingly, the included chapters reflect these foci and associated 'hands on' strategies. The use of text boxes provide practical tips about what to do in commonly encountered situations and give handy, practical quick guides for practice. Revised and extended appendices serve as an aide-mémoire or checklist for quick reference in relation to, among other things, tips about how to survive clinical placement, what roles health professionals have in the workplace, and a brief guide to help consumers manage medication. Extensive web-based resources provide the latest bibliography of reliable electronic resources for ease of access.

In writing this book the aim is to 'cut to the core' in terms of which practical, do-able and helpful strategies would be of use to health professionals who don't have formal mental health qualifications. I trust that readers will find this book to be a vital, practical and useful adjunct to their professional practice.

Deb O'Kane

CONTENTS

AUTHOR/REVIEWER

Author

Deb O'Kane (RMN, ENB 603, CMHN, Grad Dip Clinical Nursing, MA (Nursing), Grad Cert Higher Ed.) is a Senior Lecturer at Flinders University, Adelaide, SA, Australia. Her career has spanned the UK and Australia with a distinct focus on promoting mental health practice by collaborating with service users, carers and providers, and fostering research partnerships. Deb has a particular interest in the mental health of children and young people after working for several years in this area. She currently delivers training in undergraduate and postgraduate mental health nursing.

Reviewer

Rebecca Langman BPsychSc, BMA (University of South Australia)
Coordinator Consumer Engagement – Mental Health Clinical Program,
Central Adelaide Local Health Network (CALHN), Department for Health and Wellbeing, SA Health, Government of South Australia, Australia.

ACKNOWLEDGEMENT

In completing this fourth edition of *Mental Health: A pocket guide*, there are three people whose contributions must be acknowledged. Eimear Muir-Cochrane, Patricia Barkway and Debra Nizette wrote the first three editions and I pay tribute to their work, experience and generosity in trusting me to continue their voice and advocacy for modern mental health practices.

1

MENTAL HEALTH: EVERY HEALTH PROFESSIONAL'S BUSINESS

INTRODUCTION

If physical health is a desirable state, so too is mental health. Just as people strive for good physical health, good mental health or mental wellbeing is a core component of overall health that in turn allows us to function and live a full and meaningful life. Statements such as *no health without mental health*, first coined in the late nineties, has been a major influence for policymakers the world over, raising mental health awareness, reducing the health disparity between physical and mental illness, and ultimately helping to develop ongoing mental health reform. This chapter explores the definition of health, mental health and mental illness. It explores the impact of mental health problems and the common misconceptions that can lead to stigma and discrimination. It presents statistics on the incidence of mental illness in the community and the impact this can have on consumers, families and carers.

HEALTH, MENTAL HEALTH AND MENTAL ILLNESS

The World Health Organization (WHO) defines health as 'a state of complete physical, mental and social well-being and not merely the absence of disease or infirmity', though it has been recognised that such a statement is not sufficient to address the complexity of defining health since it implies a person cannot be truly healthy unless they have a sense of complete wellbeing (WHO 2019a). For example, if a person experiences a mental illness does this mean they cannot live a fulfilling life? Over the years, various theorists have debated the concept of health with the WHO revising their definition to encompass a broader perspective of health as 'a resource for everyday life, not the objective of living. Health is a positive concept emphasizing social and personal resources, as well as physical capacities' (WHO 2019a). This then raises the question: how is this different from mental health and mental illness?

Mental health

The term 'mental health' is synonymous with other terms such as 'mental wellbeing' or 'emotional health'. It is a term frequently used by professionals and while there is no universally accepted definition, most would agree there are common characteristics in each. According to the WHO mental health is:

> the well-being and effective functioning of individuals. It is more than the absence of a mental disorder; it is the ability to think, learn, and understand one's emotions and the reactions of others. Mental health is a state of balance, both within and with the environment.
>
> (WHO 2021)

In other words, a person's mental health is a positive concept that will affect the way they think, feel and act throughout all stages of their life from childhood onwards. Terms such as 'healthy ageing' or 'optimal ageing' have emerged in the past decade to reflect the overall wellbeing of people across the lifespan. Just as people can look at ways to maintain their physical health, strategies can also be put in place to experience positive mental health. See Box 1.1.

Effective mental health provides the capability to establish and contribute effectively to relationships, society and communities; to adjust to psychological distress through emotional regulation, to build resilience and capacity to problem solve, to feel good about ourselves and to increase productivity (work) and enjoy life. Everyone has mental health. It will fluctuate depending on what's happening in a person's life and environment. It is best to see a person's mental state as being on

---

Box 1.1   **Strategies to support mental health**

- Keep active and exercise.
- Build relationships.
- Get plenty of sleep.
- Avoid or minimise drug use.
- Identify personal strengths.
- Develop stress management and mindfulness.
- Do things that make you feel good.
- Seek help.

a continuum rather than a static state that is either good or bad. Most people will move back and forth along this continuum throughout their lives, therefore mental health problems can emerge as a response to everyday stresses when a person is not coping or is struggling to manage their thoughts, feelings and behaviour. Mental health problems are common and vary in degree of severity with more enduring and serious problems diagnosed as mental illness.

Mental illness

Mental illness, sometimes referred to as a mental disorder, can vary in severity and duration. It is defined as the presence of cognitive, affective and/or behavioural symptoms which are persistent and pervasive and impair the individual's functioning. Mental illness is like any other health problem. It can occur to anyone at any time. It covers a range of conditions where the impact of the symptoms is clinically significant and can be diagnosed according to standard criteria. Historically it was thought that a person diagnosed with a mental illness could not have 'good' mental health. Contemporary theories such as the recovery model (see Chapter 2) have since challenged this idea by seeing mental health as a separate entity that can work independently from mental illness; thus, it is possible for a person to live with a mental illness but still have positive mental health. Similarly, one may experience poor mental health but not have a mental health problem or mental illness.

Experiencing a mental illness is not only associated with personal attributes but is also influenced by social determinants such as poverty, education level, marital status, culture, environment and political factors, which can all contribute to the risk of mental illness (Alegría et al 2018, WHO 2019b).

STIGMA AND DISCRIMINATION

Mental health is integral to health and wellbeing, yet throughout the world mental illness is stigmatised and remains a significant health, social and human rights concern. Despite the public being more aware of mental health issues because of recent education campaigns, social media and increasing mental health awareness, attitudes from both the general population and from professionals towards people experiencing mental illness still tend to be negative. Such stigma, whether social or internalised, can contribute to poorer health outcomes for a variety of reasons, such as delayed treatment, inappropriate care, lack of services and harassment. Mental health stigma is not new and is widespread globally. Ignorance, uninformed opinions, misunderstanding often perpetuated by inaccurate information, such as media portrayal of mental illness, leads to prejudice (negative attitudes) and discrimination (prejudicial treatment and behaviour). Social isolation, reluctance to seek support, decreased employment opportunities and reduced hope are just a few of the effects of feeling stigmatised.

Progress to reduce mental health stigma is slowly taking place. Targeted approaches, often involving the narratives of people with a lived experience of mental illness, have been effective and are addressing the misconceptions of mental illness and help to break down common myths associated with particular types of mental illness. Similarly, continued work in media, tailored educational approaches and developing anti-discriminatory policy and legislation will help combat mental health stigma and enhance mental health literacy.

THE EXTENT OF MENTAL ILLNESS IN THE COMMUNITY

Worldwide statistics report that at any one time approximately one in seven people will experience a mental illness in their lifetime. Developed countries such as Australia, the UK and the United States, on average, report higher levels than this with 16–20% of the population living with a mental illness. Young people (aged 15–19 years) have the highest prevalence rate. This appears to be increasing (Ritchie & Roser 2018); however, it could be related to an increase in reporting and help seeking in response to the success of destigmatisation. If you add to these figures the number of the unknown, but significant, proportion of the population who are experiencing mental health problems, but don't seek help and subsequently go unreported, plus the global differences in data collection, the actual number of people living with mental illness in the community is greater than the statistics suggest.

International statistics for developed nations identify depression, anxiety disorders and substance-misuse disorders as the most common mental health issues (Rehm & Shield 2019). With an estimated 13% of the global population experiencing one or more mental health disorders, mental illness accounts for a substantial portion of the burden of all disease. It is clear mental health and illness are issues of major concern for the community in particular, for governments, healthcare services, non-government organisations, families, carers, friends and those people who are living with mental illness.

Having a deeper understanding of mental health, mental illness and consumers' experiences will support health professionals to deliver tailored care approaches, including the recognition of mental illness and knowing when to refer on to the appropriate services for additional support.

Vulnerable populations and individuals

Mental illness can affect anyone; however, some populations are at increased risk. At-risk populations include people who are: poor; Indigenous; from culturally and linguistically diverse backgrounds; lesbian, gay, bisexual, trans, intersex or queer (LGBTIQ); homeless; socially isolated; young men; in the justice system; victims of child abuse and domestic violence; or living with pain or a chronic illness. They also include people who have: an intellectual disability; a family history of mental illness; experienced trauma, such as refugees; chronic physical illness or comorbid drug and alcohol problems.

Despite being at increased risk, these populations often have less than optimal engagement with healthcare services. Identifying vulnerable individuals and populations who are at risk assists policymakers to plan and deliver prevention and early intervention programs to help facilitate recovery.

RISK FOR CO-OCCURRING MENTAL ILLNESS AND PHYSICAL ILLNESS

People living with a chronic physical illness are at increased risk of developing depression, anxiety and substance abuse. Comparably, people who experience mental illness die younger—10–32 years earlier than the general population. They also have higher rates of physical illness, have poorer dental health, are less likely to engage in exercise, and smoke tobacco at twice the rate of the general population (WHO 2018).

This is of concern because such disabling conditions can diminish a person's quality of life, lead to poor control of the co-occurring condition, and add to the cost of healthcare due to reduced engagement in managing the chronic health condition.

Despite these discrepancies, people with mental illness are less likely to receive hospital treatment than are the general population. For example, people who are diagnosed with schizophrenia or major depression have a 40–60% greater chance of premature death than the rest of the population, as a consequence of physical health problems that are not addressed. This is further compounded by a low level of engagement with healthcare services for this population, which in turn hinders recovery.

Social determinants—such as inequities in a person's social, physical and economic environments—also contribute to poorer health outcomes (WHO 2019b). (See Chapter 11 on co-occurring medical problems.)

IMPACT OF MENTAL ILLNESS

The impact of mental illness can be far reaching. For some people there is no significant effect, whereas for others it can have implications for employment, relationships, financial status, physical health, and education. Each person has different needs, strengths and resources that will support them in their recovery. Central to this is a person's support systems such as their family, friends and community. The ripple effect of living with someone and caring for a person with mental illness and the level of burden associated with this is well documented. Reactions to caring for a loved one may vary dependent on the seriousness of the illness, the resilience and coping styles of the caregiver, availability of support, gender and age.

Caring for a person with mental illness can be challenging, leading to high levels of stress and fatigue resulting in both physical and mental health complications of their own. The nature of caring has largely gone unnoticed until recently, yet carers make up a large proportion of an unpaid healthcare workforce saving governments billions of dollars each year (Diminic et al 2019). Many countries such as Australia, New Zealand and the UK have recognised the important role carers play in a person's recovery and commenced looking at support mechanisms and reforms to support the needs of not only consumers but carers, too. This is particularly important when considering the needs of children who have a parent with mental illness.

Health professionals can help by being cognisant of family members and others who may be involved in care, and deliver compassionate, proficient, people-centred care for all.

PROVIDING HEALTH CARE FOR PEOPLE WITH MENTAL ILLNESS IN THE PRIMARY CARE SETTING

Most people living with mental illness live in the community, and their first point of contact with the healthcare system is usually through primary care services. Health professionals can play a key role in supporting the mental health of people living with ongoing physical conditions, such as chronic pain, terminal illness or progressive neurological disorders. Screening tools used to identify psychosocial distress can easily be administered in health centres, clinics and other primary care settings. Some are also

Box 1.2	Providing general healthcare for people with mental illness in the primary care setting

- Ask about current wellbeing and listen!
- Promote healthy lifestyle choices (healthy eating, fitness, moderate alcohol consumption).
- Undertake psychosocial assessment through the use of screening tools and review regularly.
- Screen for alcohol and drug use.
- Provide education to support healthy choices.
- Regularly review psychiatric medications and their metabolic risk.
- Establish and monitor the person's body mass index, weight, waist circumference, cholesterol levels, blood pressure and blood glucose, and respond early to any changes.
- Offer assistance to help navigate the healthcare system if required.
- Arrange specialist assessment if indicated.

available as an app on smartphones or online. These tools do not diagnose mental illness but provide opportunity for health practitioners to discuss the outcomes of the assessment and plan the next step. Hence, health professionals are ideally placed to screen for symptoms of mental illness or mental health problems in people living with chronic physical conditions and to refer for specialist assessment if indicated.

General practitioners, pharmacists and practice nurses are particularly well positioned to screen and respond to the physical health problems of people living with enduring mental illness, to promote wellbeing and to monitor for early signs of possible health issues. See Box 1.2. Physical and mental comorbidities often go undetected by many professionals as it is not regarded within their role. To successfully meet all the health needs of a person, services should be working in an integrated, coordinated and effective manner.

CONCLUSION

To rephrase and expand on the WHO slogans—not only is there *no health without mental health* but there is also *no mental health without physical health*. Furthermore, this makes *mental health every health professional's business*. By providing opportunity for people to define for themselves what is 'good health', health professionals can work effectively and in partnership with people experiencing mental health issues. Furthermore, both the acute hospital and the primary care sectors are particularly well placed to undertake the role of regular monitoring and thereby promote mental wellbeing, to prevent mental illness and to screen and intervene early when mental illness symptoms are evident—and also to respond early to physical health problems experienced by people living with mental illness.

REFERENCES

Alegría, M., NeMoyer, A., Falgàs Bagué, I., et al. (2018). Social determinants of mental health: where we are and where we need to go. *Current Psychiatry Reports*, *20*(11), 95.

Diminic, S., Hielscher, E., Harris, M. G., et al. (2019). A profile of Australian mental health carers, their caring role and service needs: results from the 2012 Survey of Disability, Ageing and Carers. *Epidemiology and Psychiatric Sciences, 28*(6), 670–681.

Rehm, J., & Shield, K. D. (2019). Global burden of disease and the impact of mental and addictive disorders. *Current Psychiatry Reports*, 21(2), 10.

Ritchie H., & Roser, M. (2018) Mental health. Online. Available. https://ourworldindata.org/mental-health 28 Jan 2021.

World Health Organization (WHO) (2018). *Guidelines for the management of physical health conditions in adults with severe mental disorders.* Geneva: World Health Organization.

World Health Organization (WHO) (2019a). Definition of health. Online. Available: https://www.publichealth.com.ng/world-health-organizationwho-definition-of-health/ 28 Jan 2021.

World Health Organization (WHO) (2019b). Mental disorders. Online. Available: https://www.who.int/news-room/fact-sheets/detail/mental-disorders 28 Jan 2021.

World Health Organization (WHO) (2021). Mental health. Online. Available: https://www.who.int/westernpacific/health-topics/mental-health 21 April 2021.

WEB RESOURCES

Australian College of Mental Health Nurses, Chronic disease and mental health: http://www.acmhn.org/chronic-disease-elearning. This is a free interactive e-learning program for nurses working with people who live with chronic disease. It uses video vignettes and a range of activities to highlight the key issues related to mental health.

Australian Government, Department of Health and Ageing: https://www1.health.gov.au/internet/main/publishing.nsf/Content/mental-fifth-national-mental-health-plan. This is the site for the *Fifth National Mental Health Plan: an agenda for collaborative government action in mental health 2017–2022*.

Mental Health Foundation United Kingdom: https://www.mentalhealth.org.uk/our-work. A site with various publications, statistics and resources relevant to mental health.

Mental Health Foundation New Zealand: https://www.mentalhealth.org.nz/. The foundation works to enhance and ensure the mental health of all New Zealanders. The site provides resources and information about mental health and illness for the general public and health professionals, including links to mental healthcare services.

National Institute of Mental Health: https://www.nimh.nih.gov/health/statistics/mental-illness.shtml. This is a site providing information on mental health to improve the understanding and health of all Americans. It provides resources such as statistics, fact sheets and policy development.

World Health Organization: https://www.who.int/teams/mental-health-and-substance-use. This site has many resources with an emphasis on prevention, promotion, treatment, rehabilitation, care and recovery. The site is global in scope and aims to provide guidance for national action plans.

2 WORKING IN A RECOVERY FRAMEWORK

INTRODUCTION

A recovery-oriented approach to mental healthcare aims to facilitate mental health, minimise the impact of mental illness and manage the symptoms of mental illness. The recovery model emerged in the latter part of the 20th century amid worldwide reform of mental health services. It is a person-centred approach underpinned by principles of social justice and equity, which challenges an exclusive biomedical model of focusing mainly on symptom identification and treatment. This chapter examines the principles of recovery as a framework within which to deliver mental health services from the perspective of people with mental illness and their carers, health professionals and the healthcare system.

RECOVERY

Most people when thinking about the term 'recovery' tend to assume recovery is returning to a state of health prior to illness, injury or disease. This is often referred to as *clinical recovery*. Recovery in mental healthcare, however, is a practical approach and a philosophy of care that embraces individual strengths, resources and resilience. It incorporates social justice principles with an emphasis on the person's wellbeing, autonomy and empowerment. Recovery is not just about reducing or eliminating symptoms; it is about a person's journey while living with mental illness. Recovery in this context has many meanings. It is an individual and a dynamic experience, not a static process. Anthony, an early advocate of the recovery approach, described the journey as:

> . . . a deeply personal, unique process of changing one's attitudes, values, feelings, goals, skills, and/or roles. It is a way of living a satisfying, hopeful, and contributing life even within the limitations caused by illness. Recovery involves the development of new meaning and purpose in one's life as one grows beyond the catastrophic effects of mental illness.
>
> (Anthony 1993)

For people with mental illness and for carers, therefore, recovery means living well with an ongoing mental illness, having hope and setting goals for the future—not just symptom management. It encompasses learning about the illness and factors that trigger episodes, and making necessary lifestyle changes. For health professionals, recovery means not only working with the person to manage the symptoms of mental illness but also working with the person to enable them to lead a full and meaningful life, despite the illness.

Throughout the 20th century the core focus of mental healthcare was dominated by a biomedical framework concentrating on symptom identification and reduction with less emphasis on the subjective experience. Recent decades, however, largely driven by the consumer movement have seen a shift towards a recovery approach and person-centred care, with the *phenomenon* (i.e. the lived experience of the person with mental illness) now central in mental health services. Identifying, respecting and valuing that each person will have a personal experience of mental illness empowers people to define their own journey of recovery that can then be supported by services, health professionals and organisations. Table 2.1 provides a comparison

TABLE 2.1

Comparison of biomedical and recovery-focused understandings

Biomedical approach to mental illness	Person-centred recovery approach
A linear process of illness and wellness	A cyclical process of trying and trying again
Focus on treatment and medication management	Focus on meaningful relationships and leading an 'ordinary life'
Spirituality and meaning are not viewed as important	Spirituality is important in developing meaning and understanding
Relapse is viewed as a failure	Relapse is viewed as an opportunity for growth and learning
The experience of mental illness is a negative one	The experience of recovery from a mental illness has positive aspects
The nature of mental illness is predetermined	Having a mental illness is an individual and unique process
Relinquishing roles and responsibilities is accepted	Maintaining roles and responsibilities is promoted

of biomedical and recovery-focused understandings. The guiding principles underpinning the concept of personal recovery for a person experiencing mental illness is often known as the CHIME framework. This framework (see Fig. 2.1) (see Box 2.1) includes:

- connectedness
- hope and optimism
- identity
- meaning in life
- empowerment.

PROTECTIVE AND RISK FACTORS

A recovery approach acknowledges that some factors increase the risk of relapse, while others are protective of mental health. Hence, a recovery approach encompasses more than merely treating or managing the symptoms of the illness. It includes recognition of and attention to the social and economic aspects of people's lives, as well as their mental illness or disability. Health professionals who use a recovery framework work in partnership with the person experiencing mental illness to maximise the quality of life. This reflects a person-centred approach where a working alliance is formed between consumers, family and carers, who are seen as experts in their own care, supported by health professionals who bring their own understanding and expertise. Recognising each person's contribution, knowledge and experience enables all parties to effectively work together towards recovery. (O'Kane 2020).

Rickwood and Thomas (2019) distinguish protective and risk factors for the development of and recovery from mental illness. Protective factors reduce the likelihood that a disorder will develop by reducing the *exposure* to risk, and by reducing the *effect* of risk factors for those exposed to risk. Protective factors also foster resilience in the face of adversity and moderate against the effects of stress, whereas risk factors increase the likelihood that a disorder will develop, exacerbate the burden of an existing disorder and can indicate a person's vulnerability.

Both protective and risk factors include genetic, biological, behavioural, sociocultural and demographic conditions and characteristics (Rickwood & Thomas 2019), with some factors being internal to the person, while others are external. Internal factors include genetics, disposition and intelligence, while external drivers comprise the social determinants of health related to social, economic, political and environmental factors, including the availability of opportunities in life and access to health services (WHO 2014).

The CHIME framework for personal recovery

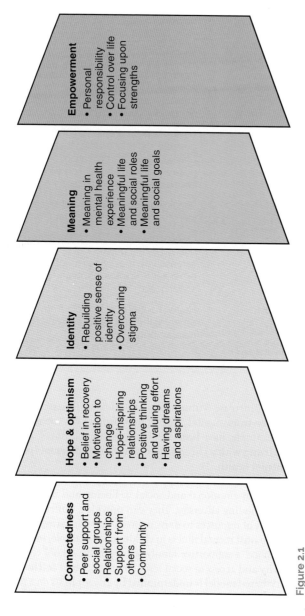

Connectedness
- Peer support and social groups
- Relationships
- Support from others
- Community

Hope & optimism
- Belief in recovery
- Motivation to change
- Hope-inspiring relationships
- Positive thinking and valuing effort
- Having dreams and aspirations

Identity
- Rebuilding positive sense of identity
- Overcoming stigma

Meaning
- Meaning in mental health experience
- Meaningful life and social roles
- Meaningful life and social goals

Empowerment
- Personal responsibility
- Control over life
- Focusing upon strengths

Figure 2.1
The CHIME framework for personal recovery
Source: Leamy et al 2011

Box 2.1	The CHIME framework for personal recovery

The CHIME framework is as follows:

Connectedness	Having good relationships and being connected to other people in positive ways. Characterised by: peer support and support groups; support from others; community.
Hope and optimism	Having hope and optimism that recovery is possible and relationships that support this. Characterised by: motivation to change; positive thinking and valuing success; having dreams and aspirations.
Identity	Regaining a positive sense of self and identity and overcoming stigma.
Meaning	Living a meaningful and purposeful life, as defined by the person (not others). Characterised by: meaning in mental 'illness experience'; spirituality; meaningful life and social goals.
Empowerment	Having control over life, focusing on strengths, and taking personal responsibility.

Source: Leamy et al 2011

Risk factors increase vulnerability to mental illness and mitigate against recovery from mental illness. Risk factors for mental illness in children, for example, have been identified as: homelessness; poor family functioning; living with a chronic illness, and poor parental (particularly maternal) mental health.

Protective factors, such as supportive family and friends, assist the person to maintain emotional and social wellbeing and to cope with life experiences—including adversity. They can provide a buffer against stress, as well as be a set of resources to draw upon to deal with stress. Factors that are protective against mental illness in children, for example, include having personal resilience, a supportive family, a supportive school environment, physical activity and access to social resources (Rickwood & Thomas 2019)

A recovery-based model is underpinned by an emphasis on a number of protective factors that can be harnessed to reduce the severity and impact of the experience of mental illness. Protective factors serve a number of purposes. They can provide a buffer against negative effects and may interrupt the processes through which risk factors operate. For example, a literacy program for illiterate young people may interrupt a potential path to unemployment. Protective factors are social determinants of health outcomes and can be grouped into three areas: individual; family and peers; and community (see Box 2.2).

RECOVERY-ORIENTED MENTAL HEALTH SERVICES

Recovery-oriented services are a fundamental component to the delivery of care in primary and hospital care. The priority is to deliver care in a

---

Box 2.2   **Protective factors**

Individual

- Resilient characteristics such as effective coping skills and being able to manage stress
- A sense of one's own spirituality
- Effective interpersonal skills
- Problem-solving skills
- A perception of social support from family and peers
- A healthy sense of self and a sense of belonging
- Positive expectations (optimism for the future)
- Meaningful activities in which to engage

Family and peers

- Good relationships and regular contact with family members
- A stable family environment with positive peer-group activities and norms
- Friends to socialise with

Community

- An economically sustainable community
- A safe and health-promoting environment
- Active community centres
- Neighbourhood cohesion

---

manner that supports the recovery of each person. The recipient of care (consumer) is acknowledged as the expert in their own life; thus, decision making, while undertaken in collaboration with health professionals, is led and directed by the person experiencing mental illness. Frameworks to support recovery-oriented practice have been established throughout mental health services. An example can be seen in Table 2.2. The principles from such frameworks can be implemented in all healthcare settings.

Recovery-oriented language

In an area where stigma and discrimination are a huge part of everyday life, the language used by health professionals, media and the general public can greatly influence the perceptions, attitudes and beliefs about mental illness. Spoken words are powerful, therefore recovery paradigms advocate for health professionals to consider their language and to choose words that demonstrate respect, genuineness and positive regard. This, in turn, promotes a culture whereby those with a lived experience of mental illness are enabled to have a voice and are more likely to establish therapeutic relationships fostering hope and resilience. A prime example of where recovery-oriented language has been implemented effectively can be seen in mental health policy and mental health reform where the term 'patient' has been replaced with consumer, service user or recipient. The latter terms reflect a person with rights, and being actively involved in any decisions concerning their health and wellbeing, whereas the term 'patient' conjures up a person who is passive in their care and takes no part in decision making.

PROVIDING RECOVERY-ORIENTED MENTAL HEALTHCARE

Hildegard Peplau first drew attention to the pivotal role of the therapeutic relationship in mental healthcare by identifying the foundation for developing a therapeutic relationship with people with mental illness as requiring unconditional positive regard, authenticity, genuineness and respect (Peplau 1952). Peplau's model also empowers health professionals 'to move away from a disease orientation to one whereby the psychological meaning of events, feelings and behaviours could be incorporated in [healthcare] interventions' (Peplau 1996).

In clinical practice, establishing rapport and a therapeutic relationship between the healthcare worker and the person with mental illness and their family is the cornerstone of effective mental healthcare. It requires

TABLE 2.2
Framework for recovery

Domain	Core principles to facilitate recovery
Promoting a culture of hope	Promote values of hope, self-determination, personal agency, social inclusion and choice. Enable a culture of hope and optimism, and encourage the person's recovery efforts.
Promoting autonomy and self-determination	Involve the person as a partner in their mental healthcare, ensuring their lived experience and expertise is recognised. Encourage informed risk taking within a safe and supportive environment, and organise the service environment to ensure safety and optimal wellbeing.
Collaborative partnerships and meaningful engagement	Provide personalised mental healthcare through collaborative partnerships with the person and their support networks. Promote mental health, wellbeing and recovery by establishing and sustaining a collaborative partnership with the person.
Focus on strengths	Focus on the person's strengths, resources, skills and assets. Support the person to build their confidence, strengths, resourcefulness and resilience.
Holistic and personalised care	Provide personalised mental healthcare informed by the person's circumstances, preferences, goals and needs. Understand the range of factors that can impact on the person's wellbeing.
Family, carers, support people and significant others	Recognise the role of family and significant others in supporting the person's recovery. Support the person to utilise and enhance their existing support networks.
Community participation and citizenship	Foster positive relationships, meaningful opportunities and community participation. Recognise the impact of stigma on recovery.
Responsiveness to diversity	Provide mental healthcare that is personalised, respectful, relevant and responsive to diversity including the person's culture and community background, gender and sexual identity.
Reflection and learning	Engage in ongoing critical reflection and continuous learning. Recognise that the person's lived experience of mental illness and recovery are valuable resources.

Source: Adapted from Department of Health 2011

empathy, trust and effective communication. The purpose of the relationship is to:

- engage with the person in order to complete a full assessment and care plan
- encourage the person to define their problems and perceptions of their distress
- facilitate the development of learning and coping skills by the person
- resolve or minimise existing problems or symptoms.

The role of health professionals in mental health promotion is to:

- facilitate a healthy lifestyle through education about diet and nutrition, rest, sleep and exercise
- support people to access employment services, housing, education and health services
- provide mental healthcare early and provide continuing intervention programs.

Peplau's model led to a shift in practice from *doing* to *being with* a person experiencing mental illness—an approach to mental healthcare that is evident in the contemporary recovery models of today, such as the Tidal Model, an approach underpinned by the core value of the consumer being central in care. This includes empowering the consumer to reclaim their personal story of mental distress in order to reclaim their lives, and the role of health professionals to help people realise what they want in relation to their lives.

WORKING WITH INDIVIDUALS

When working with individuals to facilitate recovery, Rethink (the leading United Kingdom mental health charity) challenges an exclusive biomedical model approach of focusing on illness and symptom management, advocating a model in which *mental wellness* is the goal. Rethink recommends an approach that:

- focuses on goals, not problems
- values the strengths the person brings to their personal recovery
- respects the person's self-direction
- creates an environment that supports personal recovery and values small steps (Rethink 2017).

In summary, the Rethink model is *person-centred* and directed, and proposes working with the person's strengths and addressing issues of everyday living—as well as managing the symptoms of mental illness and respecting the person's dignity of risk (i.e. enabling choices through facilitating autonomy and self-determination).

RECOVERY ACROSS THE LIFESPAN

Most of the literature and research on the concept of mental health recovery has been focused on adults. That is not to say that recovery-oriented care is not applicable for infants, children, young people or seniors. As already established, recovery is relative and different for everyone. The principles of recovery are flexible. They can be applied and adapted to reflect each individual's needs as they move across the lifespan. Aspects such as developmental issues, identity formation, psychosocial conflict, and autonomy versus dependence can all influence a child or young person's perception of their recovery journey (Law et al 2020). Related to this is the perception of health professionals who may inadvertently disregard the voice of a young person in favour of their careers. Health professionals can support children and young people to build resilience, identify prevention strategies and assist in achieving their developmental goals.

Similarly, there can be a misconception that it is futile implementing recovery approaches for older adults including people with dementia and yet contemporary research has identified working within a recovery framework is just as important. There may be additional challenges to consider such as physical decline, loss of income, loss of support networks, but being able to maintain their identity, continuing to have agency within their life and sustaining social support are fundamental to delivering a recovery-oriented approach when working with older adults (NSW Ministry of Health 2018).

WORKING WITH FAMILIES AND CARERS

Recognising the important role family and carers play in the care and recovery of a person is necessary to truly reflect recovery-oriented healthcare. They are key people to form partnerships with when delivering recovery-oriented care. Recovery-oriented approaches should support and educate families and carers to build on their strength and resilience to enhance their lives. Offering recovery-related educational courses and peer support groups can develop a stronger voice for families in the mental health and addiction system, and raise awareness of issues from a family perspective. More recently, carers have been acknowledged as key stakeholders of mental health services (e.g. as members of advisory committees and boards) in policy development, in service roles such as carer consultants and in the development of curriculum and delivery of education.

Addressing the needs of families and caregivers acknowledges the significant role they play in caregiving and, importantly, that they too have needs as a consequence of their caregiving role. See Box 2.3.

> **Box 2.3** Promoting recovery when working with families and carers
>
> - Take interest in family and caregivers.
> - Make family and carers feel welcome; for example, orientate them to the environment.
> - Provide information and resources to educate the family and carers.
> - Include family and carers in decision making whenever possible.
> - Recognise and identify the family's strengths and resources.
> - Keep discussions open and transparent and be prepared to answer any questions.
> - Discuss what family and carers understand about mental illness and recovery.
> - Explore strategies to support recovery.
> - Discuss a family or carer's own wellbeing and assist with resourcing help if required, such as respite.
> - Refer the family to a carer consultant, peer-support group or other service that may offer support and assistance.

RECOVERY COMPETENCIES FOR HEALTH WORKERS

Recovery-oriented care requires healthcare professionals to have the appropriate skills and competencies to ensure effective care is being delivered. The former New Zealand Mental Health Commissioner Mary O'Hagan describes a competent worker in the area of mental health as one who:

> understands recovery principles and experiences, supports service users' personal resourcefulness, accommodates diverse views on mental health issues, has self-awareness and respectful communication skills, protects service users' rights, understands discrimination and how to reduce it, can work with diverse cultures, understands and supports the user/survivor movement, and understands and supports family perspectives.

(O'Hagan 2004, p. 2)

You do not need to be a specialist in mental health in order to deliver competent care. Most professionals working in health or social care will at some point in their life, if not daily, encounter people experiencing mental health issues. As mental health providers, understanding the principles of recovery, supporting people on their own journey by recognising diversity, considering the strengths and resourcefulness of each person, working in partnerships with consumers and carers and being self-aware enough to identify personal values, attitudes and limitations is an excellent starting point.

RECOVERY AND RISK

When working within a recovery framework (which encourages individual choice, empowerment and self-management), tensions can arise regarding risk management. Accepting that a level of risk tolerance is required, balanced with a professional's duty of care when appraising risk and making decisions known to oppose a person's wishes can be difficult. An honest and transparent team approach, inclusive of the consumer, family and carers allows for decisions to be made with consultation and negotiation allowing for choice and self-determination to remain pivotal in a person's recovery.

Increasing in popularity as a way to foster recovery is the concept of 'positive risk taking'. Positive and therapeutic risk taking involves open dialogue between all parties with the intention of a person making decisions about their personal safety and, if mistakes are made (as inevitably they will be on occasion), they are discussed and evaluated, allowing all those involved to reflect and learn from the situation. As professionals, the role may include:

- assisting the person to decide what is an appropriate level of risk taking for their recovery within the limits of duty of care
- balancing the risk by articulating the threshold of risk that is appropriate for the setting and within the parameters of duty of care
- providing guidance, training and support to staff regarding flexible responses to a person's circumstances and preferences while maintaining appropriate risk management (Young et al 2015).

CONCLUSION

Recovery is the journey undertaken by the person living with mental illness (often in collaboration with a health professional) as the person *rethinks* their identity, goals and hopes (Slade 2013). For health professionals, practising within a recovery framework involves working with the person and their family to understand the person's story/narrative, identify strengths, set goals and address issues of everyday living—as well as managing the symptoms of mental illness.

Finally, as a guiding framework for clinical practice, recovery is an approach to achieving *mental health*, which involves more than the absence of symptoms of mental illness. It includes notions of hope and empowerment of people with mental illness and their carers, the delivery of person-centred care and the establishment of a partnership between people with mental illness, carers and health professionals in attaining the goal of mental health. Importantly, there is a focus on the person's strengths rather than the deficits that may be a consequence of the mental illness.

REFERENCES

Anthony, W. (1993). Recovery from mental illness: the guiding vision of the mental health service system in the 1990s. *Psychosocial Rehabilitation Journal, 16*(4), 11–23.

Department of Health. (2011). Framework for recovery-oriented practice. Melbourne: Mental Health, Drug and Alcohol Division, State Government of Victoria.

Law, H., Gee, B., Dehmahdi, N., et al. (2020). What does recovery mean to young people with mental health difficulties? – 'It's not this magical unspoken thing, it's just recovery'. *Journal of Mental Health, 29*(4), 464–472. Online. Available: http://www.hdc.org.nz/publications/other-publications-from-hdc/mental-health-resources/recovery-competencies-for-new-zealand-mental-health-workers 15 July 2017.

Leamy, M., Bird, V., Le Boutillier, C., et al. (2011). Conceptual framework for personal recovery in mental health: systematic review and narrative synthesis. *British Journal of Psychiatry, 199*(6), 445–452.

NSW Ministry of Health (2018). *NSW Older People's Mental Health Recovery-oriented Practice Improvement Project: statewide project report.* NSW Health: Sydney.

O'Hagan, M. (2004). Recovery in New Zealand: lessons for Australia? Guest editorial. *Australian e-Journal for the Advancement of Mental Health, 3*(1), 1–3.

O'Kane, D. (2020). Partnerships in health. In P. Barkway & D. O'Kane (Eds.), *Psychology: an introduction for health professionals.* Sydney: Elsevier.

Peplau, H. (1952). *Interpersonal relations in nursing.* New York: GP Putnam.

Peplau, H. (1996). Fundamental and special—the dilemma of psychiatric and mental health nursing. *Commentary Archives of Psychiatric Nursing, 10*(1), 14–15.

Rethink. (2017). Recovery. Online. Available: http://www.rethink.org/living-with-mental-illness/recovery 5 February 2021.

Rickwood, D.J. & Thomas, K.A. (2019). Mental wellbeing interventions: an Evidence Check rapid review brokered by the Sax Institute (https://www.saxinstitute.org.au/) for VicHealth.

Slade, M. (2013). *100 ways to support recovery: a guide for mental health professionals* (2nd ed.). London: Rethink Recovery Series. Online. Available: https://www.rethink.org/media/704895/100_ways_to_support_recovery_2nd_edition.pdf 5 February 2021.

World Health Organization (WHO) (2014). Social determinants of mental health. Online. Available: http://apps.who.int/iris/bitstream/10665/112828/1/9789241506809_eng.pdf 10 February 2021.

Young, A.T., Green, C.A., Estroff, S.E. (2015) New endeavors, risk-taking, and personal growth in the recovery process: findings from the STARS study. *Psychiatric Services, 59,* 1430–1436.

WEB RESOURCES

Choices in Recovery: https://www.choicesinrecovery.com/mental-health-recovery. html. A site to support people living with schizophrenia and schizoaffective disorder to grow the confidences and skills needed to meet the challenges of daily life.

Embrace CareGivers: https://embracecaregivers.com/en/. A Canadian site developed by caregivers, health professionals and services offering education, resources and information to family and care givers.

Emerge Aotearoa: https://emergeaotearoa.org.nz/about-us/our-history/. Emerge Aotearoa was formed by the merging of Recovery Solutions (formerly Carnegie Trust) and the Richmond Fellowship. It promotes mental health and recovery for people living with mental illness by providing culturally appropriate, community-based rehabilitation within an accommodation support framework for people living with mental illness or addiction and drug abuse.

Recovery Hub: http://recovery.awh.org.au. Recovery Hub contains many activities, articles and practical resources to provide choice, encourage hope and inspire people with mental illness to improve their health and wellness and to live a positive lifestyle.

Recovery Oriented Language Guide: https://mhcc.org.au/wp-content/uploads/ 2019/08/Recovery-Oriented-Language-Guide_2019ed_v1_20190809-Web. pdf. This document offers guidelines for professionals to support them in communication using recovery-oriented language.

Rethink (UK): www.rethink.org. Rethink is the largest charity in the UK supporting severe mental illness. It is dedicated to improving the lives of everyone affected by severe mental illness, whether they have a condition themselves, care for others who do, or are professionals or volunteers working in the mental health field.

Tidal Model: www.tidal-model.com. The Tidal Model is the first mental health recovery model developed *conjointly* by mental health nurses and people who have used mental health services.

3

ESSENTIALS FOR MENTAL HEALTH PRACTICE

INTRODUCTION

People seeking assistance for mental health concerns require care that meets their needs for support, treatment, information, advocacy or refuge. All care delivered by health professionals needs to be generated from values such as respect and concern for each person and their experience. Values-based care guides the provision of appropriate healthcare and promotes the connection between the healthcare provider and the person seeking support.

For health professionals from all disciplines, their level of education and unique discipline knowledge, personal values and established standards and principles of practice guide them in their practice. This chapter outlines some key components of practice when working with people needing mental healthcare.

The chapter introduces the term 'working alliance' to establish that health professionals work with people with mental illness in a committed professional partnership, acknowledging their experience and supporting the person's recovery (see Chapter 2).

Mental health promotion and prevention of mental illness underpin mental healthcare. Promotion and prevention aim to strengthen a person's resilience. They aim to increase protective factors and lessen a person's vulnerability to mental health problems. For those who are unwell, promotion and prevention strategies aim to increase relapse-prevention skills. A focus on individual strengths and building resilience are a necessary component of recovery-oriented practice.

PRACTICE ESSENTIALS
Practice standards

Mental health conditions are global and widespread and yet in certain countries, psychiatrists or other mental healthcare-trained providers are scarce. Poor-quality services and lack of trained professionals can result in unrecognised mental health problems, human rights violations and poor treatment outcomes. While some countries have established services that reflect best practice and continue to improve the quality of care being delivered, other countries do not have the capacity to do this and people using services are often exposed to long admissions, being detained without informed consent and subject to harmful practice. The World Health Organization (WHO) in identifying these discrepancies has set a goal that by 2023, 100 million people will have access to appropriate and affordable mental healthcare (WHO 2019).

In response to the needs of people with mental health conditions, a number of countries have developed guidelines, often referred to as standards, to describe the care required to promote recovery. Such standards may consist of ethical and professional guidelines that are not mandated but provide a supporting framework for high-quality mental health practice, whereas others are legislative in nature. For instance, there are 13 national practice standards that relate to all health professionals working with people with mental illness and their families in Australia. The standards aim to provide a benchmark for practice, education and skill development. Table 3.1 lists the 13 practice standards. Other practice standards have been developed to cover specific population groups; for example, youth, aged care and intellectual disability, which are applicable to all professionals delivering mental healthcare regardless of their discipline and background.

Guiding principles

The following principles form the basis for a holistic, preventative, health-promoting and recovery-oriented system of specialised care (Department of Health 2013). The guiding principles below are embedded in the Standards (Table 3.1).

- Promote an ideal quality of life for people with a mental illness.
- Supply services with the aim of facilitating sustained recovery for people with a mental illness.
- Involve service users in all decisions regarding their treatment, support and care, including the option to choose their treatment and setting if possible.
- Acknowledge the right of the person to have their nominated carer involved in all aspects of their care and treatment.
- Recognise the role played by carers, including their needs and require-ments, which is separate from the person receiving treatment.
- Learn about the people and carers using the service, in order to value their lived experiences.

TABLE 3.1
National practice standards for the mental health workforce 2013

National standard	Explanation (adapted from the practice standards overview)
1. Rights, responsibilities, safety and privacy	Mental health professionals uphold the rights of people affected by mental health problems and mental disorders, and those of their family members or carers, maintaining their privacy, dignity and confidentiality, and actively promoting their safety.
2. Working with people, families and carers in recovery-focused ways	Mental health professionals support people to become decision makers in their own care.
3. Meeting diverse needs	Mental health professionals respectfully respond to the social, cultural, linguistic, spiritual and gender diversity of people with mental illness and of carers, incorporating those differences in their practice.
4. Working with Aboriginal and Torres Strait Islander people, families and communities	Mental health professionals provide culturally safe systems of care, reduce barriers to access and improve social and emotional wellbeing.
5. Access	Mental health professionals facilitate timely access to quality evidence-based assessment.
6. Individual planning	Mental health professionals facilitate and support care planning from a quality evidence base.
7. Treatment and support	Mental health professionals provide quality evidence-informed interventions.
8. Transitions in care	Mental health professionals support the exit or transition of a person's care in a structured and timely way.
9. Integration and partnership	Mental health professionals recognise and support the provision of coordinated care across the broad network of carers, community, programs and services.
10. Quality improvement	Mental health professionals collaborate with people with a lived experience, families and team members to actively improve mental health practices.

TABLE 3.1
National practice standards for the mental health workforce 2013—cont'd

National standard	Explanation (adapted from the practice standards overview)
11. Communication and information management	Mental health professionals establish therapeutic relationships and maintain quality documentation, information systems and evaluation to monitor and evaluate needs.
12. Health promotion and prevention	Mental health clinicians seek to build resilience in individuals and communities through mental health promotion and primary prevention principles.
13. Ethical practice and professional development responsibilities	Mental health professionals are aware of their individual scope of practice and the codes and regulations supporting their practice; they take responsibility for their own professional development and continuing education and contribute to the development of others.

Source: Adapted from Department of Health 2013

- Recognise and advocate the rights of children and young people affected by a family member with a mental illness to appropriate protection, care and information.
- Support participation and contribution by people, their families and carers as part of the mental health service development, planning, delivery and evaluation process.
- Modify mental health treatment, support and care to meet the specific needs of the individual.
- When delivering mental health treatment, aim to provide a plan that takes into account the individual's living situation, needs of their family or carer and level of support within the community to ensure the least amount of personal restriction on the individual's rights and choices.
- Implement evidence-informed practices and quality improvement processes.
- Participate in professional development activities.

More recently projects have been developed to address issues of social inclusion, stigma and discrimination with the aim to include and value people with a lived experience of mental illness and further support integration of recovery-oriented care.

Settings and models for care

The environment across mental healthcare settings is sometimes referred to as the *therapeutic milieu*. The environment is seen as being 'therapeutic' in itself if the following underlying principles are supported:

- Open communication
- Democratisation
- Orientation to the therapeutic milieu
- Privacy and respect for one another
- Group cohesion.

Mental health professionals can influence and increase the therapeutic potential of the environment by creating and promoting the following elements in the environment (Sharrock et al 2017):

- A place of safety
- A predictable, organised structure
- Personal and social support
- Involvement and collaboration in the care environment
- Validation of each person's individual experience through interpersonal communication
- Symptom management
- Maintaining links with the person's family and support structure
- Developing links and resources in the community.

More and more care is being delivered to people in their local community or their home through a range of non-government, primary health and community organisations and partnerships. Care delivered in diverse settings has seen the development of a range of models of care—for example, integrated teams that provide triage, crisis and case management and hence optimise and streamline care delivery and recovery. Another example is the Mental Health Nurse Incentive Program where credentialled mental health nurses work to their full scope of practice providing primary and supportive ongoing care to people with the full range of mental health issues.

Teamwork

The 'multidisciplinary team' is a team approach for care delivery. Because the multidisciplinary team comprises nursing, medical and allied health professionals, this model optimises options for the person, as each health professional has unique and complementary skills that provide holistic coordinated care to assist the person's recovery. There can be overlap in skill sets among mental health professionals, so frequent meetings are required to ensure coordinated care.

'Case management' is a model of care in which treatment options and care delivery is provided and coordinated by one health professional in a consistent manner. Case management can be used in all mental health settings; its strengths are that the case manager can refer the person to other members of the team with expertise to meet the person's specific needs.

Scope of practice

Each health practitioner works within a 'scope of practice', which describes the full spectrum of roles, functions, responsibilities, activities and decision-making capacity that individuals within professions are educated, competent and authorised to perform. The scope defines boundaries of responsibility and accountability for each mental health professional and therefore influences decision making in care and service delivery. Scope of practice within the multidisciplinary team requires that individual members negotiate care delivery and establish who is responsible for particular care or services according to their individual scope of practice, even if a particular discipline is accountable for care or service delivery.

MENTAL HEALTH LITERACY AND PSYCHOEDUCATION

'Mental health literacy' refers to an individual's or group's awareness, understanding and knowledge about mental health and illness. It can influence their response to recognising signs or behaviours of mental illness and identifying pathways for treatment and recovery. Mental health practitioners and people with mental illness play an important role in increasing public awareness and understanding of mental illness to facilitate early recognition and intervention.

Awareness raising and increasing mental health literacy can be achieved by identifying or providing resources such as:

- information sheets about mental health services, types of treatments and types of mental health problems
- medication information sheets (in a style and format appropriate for the general public)
- website addresses
- referrals to and engagement with community support groups, parenting programs, employment programs, abuse-related programs, addiction programs, health advisory groups and health and mental health education programs
- peer support services.

'Psychoeducation' is the provision of information required by the person, their family or a group to improve mental health literacy, self-determination and quality of life. Mental health literacy and psychoeducation are vital to enabling the person and family to determine their own needs and to make their own decisions about treatment and recovery.

ASSESSMENT

Assessment is an ongoing process because a person's functioning can change depending on what is happening in their environment (internal and external). The person's internal environment consists of their thoughts, feelings and physical health; their external environment can be their family, their physical world and the social relationships within it. A range of assessments can be performed by different mental health professionals depending on a person's presentation and needs.

Holistic mental health assessment measures the person's functioning in the following domains:

- Physical
- Cultural
- Spiritual
- Mental and emotional (mental state assessment; see Chapter 5)
- Developmental and functional
- Family
- Social/environmental.

PRACTITIONER ESSENTIALS
Personal and professional values

Humanistic and holistic values underpin the mental health practice for many health professionals. 'Humanism' can be defined as a perspective on life that is centred on a concern for human interests, values and upholding a person's dignity. It is particularly relevant in healthcare when people may be vulnerable and seeking assistance. 'Holism' in health relates to the idea that the person is more than the sum of their parts and that if we recognise the importance of the interrelationships between the biological, psychological, social and spiritual aspects of the person, healing and wellbeing are enhanced.

Important values include the following:

- A *person-centred approach.* A person-centred approach is essential for mental healthcare. You are there for the person and to liaise with carers/family/friends as appropriate.
- A *working alliance.* Developing a working alliance enables you to understand the person's (and family's) recovery plan. Work with the person to achieve recovery defined by them using their strengths. You remain positive and hopeful and support their recovery plan.

- *Compassionate care.* Compassionate care supports recovery and emotional wellbeing. It matters how you care because it affects the person and their family's feelings (e.g. maintain compassion and best practice in situations of distress, anxiety and 'busyness').
- *Respect.* Respect underpins person-centred care and includes respect for both the person and their experience.
- A *'safe' environment.* Mental healthcare is best delivered in environments that support *cultural, physical and emotional safety.* Encourage feedback about the environment and appropriateness of care delivery.
- A *multidisciplinary team.* A multidisciplinary team approach presents the person with a wide range of therapies and treatment options suitable to promote recovery.

Self-awareness and self-care

'Self-awareness' involves consciousness of our own values, beliefs, attitudes and motivations and understanding how they may affect others. It also includes the ability to reflect on and accommodate the values and beliefs of others. Self-awareness is developed over time through experience and focused activities. It requires being grounded in the here and now and knowing our thoughts, feelings and reactions. Health professionals who know their own strengths and limitations, understand how their values, attitudes and emotions can affect their communication and actions and enable a genuine presentation of oneself when working with others. Having this awareness will help you to focus on people with mental illness, families and their needs despite the times it can be challenging both on a professional and personal level. It is therefore important to not only improve levels of self-awareness but also self-care. Strategies that can develop self-awareness and constitute professional self-care include:

- clinical supervision
- mentorship
- professional development and education
- requesting feedback on your practice
- asking questions of mentors
- keeping a journal of your practice for reflection or discussion with a mentor
- debriefing.

Appendix 1 provides some guidance on surviving clinical placement and engaging in professional self-care.

As well as professional self-care, personal self-care is essential for anyone working in the human services. Engaging on a therapeutic and interpersonal level with people who are in crisis, are experiencing loss or have difficulty managing their own thoughts, feelings, emotions and behaviour can be demanding and sometimes exhausting. Recognising our own needs and developing strategies to maintain wellbeing are essential. Personal self-care requires an active awareness of our health and wellbeing needs. Self-care is any preventative and balancing activity that is activated to optimise our personal coping when we are stressed and challenged emotionally, cognitively and physically.

Strategies to promote personal self-care may include:

- physical self-care and activity—exercise such as running, yoga and sport, good nutrition, sleep hygiene
- psychological self-care—reflection, meditation and mindfulness; journalling and reading
- emotional and spiritual self-care—relaxation and social-connectedness; dancing, artistic activity, music.

Creating a plan of self-care helps protect and manage personal mental health. Learning how to recognise the first signs of stress, such as feeling unable to cope, lethargy, anxiety or no longer finding job satisfaction, can prevent a person becoming overwhelmed and burnt out in their job. Burnout is a term used to describe a state of complete physical, mental and emotional exhaustion. It occurs as a result of prolonged unresolved stress and can have a negative impact on family life, employment and health. Using self-help strategies and/or seeking professional help can help replenish personal resources and maintain wellbeing.

The working alliance

The aim of the working alliance is to develop a relationship where the therapeutic goals for the person and/or family can be realised. In this context, mental health professionals use their knowledge and their own strengths and insights (developed from professional and personal self-care) to use the 'self' as a therapeutic tool. Empathy, understanding the person's experience and working with them to achieve their goals is the process essential to the alliance. The following is a framework for the working alliance:

- Professional boundaries are in place and are the responsibility of the practitioner.
- The person with mental illness and their recovery pathway are the focus of the alliance.
- The person with mental illness determines or defines their desired outcomes of the working alliance.

- Respect for the experience of the person and a non-judgmental attitude are essential for care provision.
- Communication skills are the foundation of the working alliance. The practitioner often needs to role-model health-communication techniques.

Box 3.1 provides some tips for initiating the alliance, Box 3.2 provides tips for developing and maintaining the alliance and Box 3.3 provides tips for building strengths in the alliance.

Professional boundaries

Boundaries refer to verbal and non-verbal actions and interactions between individuals or groups of people. Safe and appropriate boundaries are in place when interactions are mutually respectful of the person or group, their culture and experience. Health practitioners are responsible for setting and/or negotiating boundaries in the working alliance to focus on and facilitate the achievement of the person's goals. Most professions have codes of conduct or codes of ethics that identify boundary setting as part of the professional responsibility. Box 3.4 provides tips for setting boundaries.

Pathways to developing expertise and the capacity to provide holistic assessment and care in mental health work exist in the professional health disciplines and human services. Acquiring additional communication, engagement and therapeutic alliance skills, as well as self-awareness, promotes the potential for the wellbeing and recovery of people with mental illness.

| **Box 3.1** | **Tips for initiating the alliance: developing rapport** |

- Put aside everything else that is happening to you and around you, and focus on the person.
- Choose a time and place to invite the person to tell you their story or to discuss their issue when it is convenient for them.
- Be gentle and confident in your approach. You may lead the interaction initially by inviting the person to set timelines. However, the person will take the lead and define their therapeutic needs.
- Collaborate with the person in setting expectations and timelines for the working alliance.

Box 3.2 | **Tips for developing and maintaining the alliance: responding**

How can you respond usefully? Everything you need to know about the person is in what they tell you and what you observe in their appearance and behaviour. Listed below are steps to a useful response.

Listen

- Listen to the person's story for content (the 'what' of their story), their feelings (the tone of their story) and themes (the priorities of their story).
- Identify a keyword, feeling or theme, and reflect it back—for example, 'You mentioned you had a car accident *(content)*. Can you tell me more about it?' 'You sounded angry *(feeling)* when you told me about your car accident.' 'You mentioned your car accident several times *(theme)*. It sounds like it was a significant event in your life.' Any of these responses, plus single-word prompts or non-verbal nods also work to indicate to the person that you are listening and interested in hearing more.

Pay attention

- Show in your body language that you are making an effort to attend to the story.
- Summarise and clarify content, feelings and themes in the person's story—for example, 'You continue to be angry and blame yourself for the car accident and it sounds like you find it difficult to cope with your anger in general since the accident. Is this how it is for you?'
- Explore previous coping and available or needed skills and options for the future. This exploration might need to occur at a later time when the person is less distressed or you may need to refer them to a more experienced practitioner. Negotiate a time for further alliance work.

Box 3.3 | **Tips for building strengths in the alliance: developing resilience**

Resilience can be developed by:

- encouraging mutual and shared learning (psychoeducation)
- providing and exploring options
- being clear and assertive

- challenging and responding openly to challenge
- identifying and providing resources
- maintaining a positive attitude
- role-modelling a wellness attitude
- persevering and maintaining hope.

Box 3.4   **Tips for setting boundaries**

- Introduce yourself and say what you prefer to be called and the purpose of your role. Consistently refer to the person using their preferred title.

- Keep a focus on the person's story during communication with the person. Keeping the storyline in focus helps them tell a rich and detailed story, free of distractions.

- Provide summaries and updates on therapeutic goals. Summaries will help the person self-monitor and keep a focus on their recovery.

- Remain open and non-judgmental. Humanistic values promote the concept of unconditional positive regard (i.e. unconditional acceptance of the person—not necessarily to any behaviours or feelings).

- Criticism or disapproval is a warning of boundary vulnerability. Attempt to clarify instead.

- Discuss any uncomfortable or unexpected feelings or feelings of confusion with your line or clinical supervisor. Feelings of guilt, anger and attraction can disrupt the alliance.

- Remember that the alliance is not the same as a social relationship. Stop and reflect if it starts to feel like friendship. This includes things friends typically do such as giving each other small gifts, making contact out of work time or chatting socially. All of these behaviours impair the alliance and are warnings of a boundary threat.

- Respond respectfully and thoughtfully to the person with mental illness at all times. Keeping your communication at a professional level will keep the alliance on track.

- Engage in clinical supervision. Clinical supervision develops your practice expertise and professional awareness.

CONCLUSION

Working from a humanistic and holistic values base is the foundation for mental health work; it also requires an awareness of and adherence to national standards/principles and any jurisdictional standards as a baseline for practice. Skill in developing the working alliance increases with experience, feedback from people with mental illness and peers, clinical supervision and greater self-awareness from critical reflection on practice. Most importantly, it is essential for the helpers to care for themselves because self-care can have a positive impact on professional quality of life.

REFERENCES

Department of Health. (2013). *National practice standards for the mental health workforce 2013.* Melbourne: State Government of Victoria.

Sharrock, J., Maude, P., Wilson, L., et al. (2017). Settings for mental health. In K. Evans, D. Nizette, & A. O'Brien (Eds.), *Psychiatric and mental health nursing* (4th ed.). Sydney: Elsevier.

World Health Organization (WHO). (2019). *Special initiative for mental health (2019–2023).* Online. Available: https://www.who.int/publications/i/item/special-initiative-for-mental-health-(2019-2023) . 10 February 2021.

WEB RESOURCES

Department of Developmental Disability Neuropsychiatry: Intellectual Disability Mental Health Core Competency Framework: https://www.3dn.unsw.edu.au/IDMH-CORE-COMPETENCY-FRAMEWORK. This framework supports health professionals to develop core competencies in the area of intellectual disability mental health.

HelpGuide: Burnout Prevention and Treatment: https://www.helpguide.org/articles/stress/burnout-prevention-and-recovery.htm. A site that offers support strategies for self-care and stress management.

Orygen: Workforce competencies for youth mental health: https://www.orygen.org.au/Training/Resources/Service-knowledge-and-development/Clinical-practice-points/Workforce-competencies-youth-mh. A document comprising the shared key skills required from a multidisciplinary team when working with young people.

WHO MiNDbank: https://www.mindbank.info/. A database promoting inclusiveness in the area of disability by providing resources in a number of areas including policy, standards of care, advocacy and human rights.

4

AN OVERVIEW OF MENTAL HEALTH PROBLEMS

INTRODUCTION

This chapter provides a quick reference to the common mental illnesses that health professionals may come across in their daily practice. Incidence, causative factors and descriptions of the major mental illnesses are covered, with reference to useful websites. The major mental illnesses include disorders of anxiety, mood, thinking and perception and personality disorders. It is increasingly recognised that the diagnostic classifications of mental illness as well as the concept of schizophrenia are inaccurate and provide an incomplete perspective of the experiences of mental illness. With this in mind, disorders specific to particular populations—the young, the elderly, those with intellectual disabilities and substance misuse disorders—are described here, acknowledging that intellectual disabilities, delirium and substance misuse disorders are not mental illnesses per se but are generally discussed in association with mental illnesses. This chapter will be of use to health professionals in the general setting where they will encounter people with physical health conditions as well as a mental health disorder, bearing in mind that diagnostic groupings can be of limited use to people with mental illness and to carers.

DIAGNOSTIC CLASSIFICATIONS

There are two main classifications for diagnosing mental illness used around the world. The 5th edition of the *Diagnostic and Statistical Manual of Mental Disorders* (known as DSM-5), which is published by the American Psychiatric Association (2013), is commonly used in most states and territories in Australia. This classification system assesses the person across five domains, which helps with treatment planning and outcomes. The *International Statistical Classification of Diseases and Related Health Problems* (ICD-11), published by the World Health Organization (2017b), provides a listing of clinical diagnoses that are coded and is commonly used in Europe and the northern hemisphere, as well as in some states of Australia (e.g. Queensland).

While there is discussion about future classification systems referring more to the experience of mental illness and specific symptoms rather than definite categories of illness such as depression and schizophrenia, these categories remain the basis of diagnosis around the world at the moment. With that in mind, it is important to note that there is significant overlap between symptoms in mood disorders and other diagnoses such as personality disorders. Further, symptoms of anxiety can occur in a range of anxiety and depressive disorders. Finally, psychotic symptoms can occur in schizophrenia, depressive and bipolar conditions. This chapter is a guide to the common mental illnesses and their symptoms but is not an exhaustive account.

AETIOLOGY OF MENTAL ILLNESS

In short, there is not enough evidence about specific theories to be certain of the causes of mental illness. There are several theories, including genetic, family history, neurochemical (imbalance of the neurotransmitter serotonin), social/cultural factors, psychological factors and upbringing. It is thought that some mental illness such as depression and schizophrenia are linked to abnormalities in many genes, not just one. In schizophrenia, for example, identical and non-identical twins are more likely to develop the disease if their twin has it (i.e. more than the general population). A person may inherit a susceptibility to a mental illness such as anxiety from one of their parents but may not necessarily develop the illness. Psychological factors include severe trauma (e.g. physical, sexual or emotional abuse), neglect and early loss of a parent.

ANXIETY AND RELATED PROBLEMS
How common?

Experiencing a level of some anxiety can be normal, particularly at times appropriate to a stressful situation; for example, before sitting an exam. Anxiety can improve a person's responsiveness by improving performance in the completion of a task. A person who experiences continuing high levels of anxiety can, however, be disabled in their thinking and functioning to an extent it impacts on daily life. Anxiety disorders around the world are widespread. The World Health Organization estimates 264 million adults live with anxiety. Of these adults, 63% are female (WHO 2017a). Anxiety is more common in people living with chronic disease, young adults and those from a Euro-Anglo background (Remes et al 2016). Most anxiety disorders develop before the age of 21 with less prevalence seen in older adults aged 60 and over.

Generalised Anxiety Disorder (GAD)

Generalised anxiety disorder is the most common anxiety disorder. It is characterised by persistent and excessive worrying for a range of situations, over a period of several months. It can occur at any time over the course of a person's life, though children and middle-aged people are at highest risk (Munir & Takov 2020). There is controversy concerning the validity of this diagnosis, with claims that such people are in fact 'the worried well' when in reality GAD can be seriously disabling and presents frequently for assistance to health services.

Symptoms

Symptoms are:

- a feeling of being consistently on edge
- excessive worry or ruminations
- fatigue
- irritability
- physical tension
- poor concentration
- restlessness.

Phobias

A phobia is defined as a marked and persistent irrational fear of something, that typically lasts more than six months. Fear is cued by the presence or anticipation of a specific object or situation (e.g. flying, heights, animals, receiving an injection, seeing blood). Exposure to the phobic stimulus results in extreme anxiety. A useful mnemonic to remember the key elements necessary for a diagnosis of phobia is 'PHOBIA':

P persistent
H handicapping (restricted lifestyle)
O object/situation
B behaviour (avoidance)
I irrational fears (recognised as such by the person)
A anxiety response.

For a diagnosis of a specific phobia, the person's fear must result in significant interference with their functioning, not just distress.

There are five subtypes of specific phobia, depending on the type of trigger. Often more than one type will be present:

- *animal:* animals or insects
- *natural environment:* for example, storms, heights and water (generally childhood onset)

- *blood/injections/injury:* seeing blood or injury, or receiving an injection or other procedure (vasovagal fainting response)
- *situational:* for example, bridges, elevators and flying
- *other:* for example, choking, vomiting and contracting an illness.

Children often experience irrational fears and this can be a normal part of childhood. More often these fears do not interfere with daily life, do not need treatment, and will disappear as a child matures, unlike adults, who, without treatment, can result in having a restricted lifestyle.

Agoraphobia

Agoraphobia is a specific fear of being in places or situations from which escape may be difficult. The term comes from the Greek *agora*, meaning marketplace, but typical agoraphobic situations include being home alone, queuing, being in a crowd or travelling on public transport.

Panic disorder

One of the main symptoms of panic disorder is to have reoccurring panic attacks that are sudden, unexpected and with no apparent cause. Anyone can have a panic attack, but this does not mean they have a panic disorder. A panic disorder is when the attacks become frequent and disabling often associated with anxiousness related to when the next attack will occur.

Obsessive-compulsive and related disorders

Anxiety is a common feature of obsessive-compulsive disorder (OCD), therefore often associated with it. While OCD may have similarities with a person experiencing anxiety there are also some distinguishing characteristics that separate it. OCD is characterised by obsessions (persistent and recurrent intrusive thoughts or feelings perceived to be inappropriate by the person) and compulsions (thoughts, actions and behaviours that the person feels compelled to undertake in order to reduce the anxiety experienced). Any reduction in anxiety is short-lived, and the obsessive thought and associated ritual compulsive behaviours recur, causing havoc in a person's daily life.

Table 4.1 lists examples of common themes of OCD.

Post-traumatic stress disorder

PTSD used to be called 'shell shock' after soldiers from World War I returned emotionally scarred from their experiences. PTSD is no longer categorised in the DSM-5 with anxiety disorders though high levels of anxiety are often inherent as one of the presenting features; it is now described under trauma and stressor-related disorders. For a diagnosis of

TABLE 4.1
Common themes of obsessive-compulsive behaviour

Obsession	Compulsion
Contamination	Excessive handwashing
Pathological doubt	Checking the gas is off or the door is locked
Physical illness	Excessive visits to a general practitioner
Need for symmetry	Lining things up, straightening things, counting or checking excessively
Religious	Excessive recitation of the rosary

PTSD, the person must have been exposed to actual or threatened death, serious injury or sexual violence.

The exposure can be:

- direct
- witnessed
- indirect, by hearing of a relative or close friend who has experienced the event—indirectly experienced death must be accidental or violent.

How common?

Incidence depends on the nature of the trauma. The prevalence of PTSD needs to be understood in the context of the prevalence of exposure to post-traumatic events (PTEs). Across their lifetime, most people (50–70%) will be exposed to a PTE and, of this group, 15–25% will develop PTSD. Prevalence of PTSD is global with 3.9% of the population experiencing it in their lifetime. This figure rises to 5.6% among those with exposure to a traumatic event. Only a minority of these go on to receive specialised treatment (Koenen et al 2017).

Symptoms

Symptoms are in four groupings focusing on the behavioural effects of symptoms, which are: intrusion; avoidance; negative alterations in cognitions and mood; and alterations in arousal and reactivity. Two new symptoms have now been added:

- persistent and distorted blame of self or others
- reckless or destructive behaviour (American Psychiatric Association 2013).

In younger children, verbalising their anxiety, reasons for avoidance or fears, may be difficult and instead their distress may be exhibited as physical complaints (e.g. head or stomach ache), mood changes or antisocial behaviour.

Treatment for anxiety disorders

Treatment involves psychological counselling with cognitive behaviour therapy being one of the most effective treatments. Applied relaxation therapy, exposure and response prevention and eye movement desensitisation therapy are other treatment options. Antidepressants also have a role in maintaining a stable mood and reducing anxiety.

SCHIZOPHRENIA
How common?

Schizophrenia is a mental illness that commonly develops between the ages of 16 and 35, affecting approximately 20 million people worldwide. It occurs equally in males and females. Schizophrenia means different things for people with the condition due to the nature of the experience of illness. For instance, there will be diverse and varying degrees of symptoms meaning that everyone's experience is unique. This may fluctuate over time with short periods of being acutely unwell to other times when a person actively engages in life, work and socialising as part of society.

People with schizophrenia will often experience episodes of psychosis. Psychosis (a symptom of schizophrenia) can be frightening as it is difficult for the person to distinguish what is real from what isn't. A distorted sense of reality can lead to unusual behaviour, thoughts and interactions with others, leaving a person feeling frightened, anxious and vulnerable.

Symptoms

Symptoms of schizophrenia include:
- delusions, hallucinations, disorganised speech, disorganised thinking (also referred to as positive symptoms)
- grossly disorganised behaviour
- flat affect, lack of volition, lack of pleasure in everyday life, diminished ability to initiate and sustain planned activity, speaking infrequently even when forced to interact (also referred to as negative symptoms).

When experiencing symptoms of schizophrenia a person may neglect basic hygiene. Health professionals can help by offering support with everyday activities and understand the impact symptoms can have to complete the activities of daily living or other tasks. Historically people with schizophrenia were seen as 'mad', 'lunatics' and 'insane' and were housed in large psychiatric facilities where barbaric treatments were a common occurrence. Today, with a better understanding of the illness and improved treatments, people can go on to to live a productive and relatively normal life.

Schizoaffective disorder

Schizoaffective disorder is characterised by the presence of symptoms of schizophrenia with an abnormal (elevated or lowered) mood.

Schizophreniform

Schizophreniform disorder differs only from the diagnosis of schizophrenia in that the duration of the symptoms is less than six months and functioning has not been negatively affected in the person.

Brief psychotic disorder

Brief psychotic disorder refers to a person experiencing a psychotic episode that endures for more than one day but less than one month. Psychosis is defined as a mental state characterised by the experience of hallucinations or delusions where the person is out of touch with reality.

Drug-induced psychosis

Drug-induced psychosis refers to a person presenting with symptoms of schizophrenia as a direct result of ingesting prescribed or non-prescribed medication.

Treatment

Treatment for schizophrenia and psychosis involves psychotropic medications, psychotherapy and psychosocial care and may be necessary for long periods. For some people where the symptoms are acute, an intensive level of care may be required such as hospitalisation or a community crisis team where recovery can take place in the least restrictive environment. While treatment is usually focused on reducing symptoms and improving the quality of life by taking medication, there is a growing number of people who choose to accept and live with their symptoms or choose a non-pharmacological approach to manage their illness and recovery.

DISORDERS OF MOOD
How common?

A mood disorder relates to the changing levels of mood in a person being either elevated or lowered. Between 3% and 5% of the global population experience depression. It is a leading cause of disability worldwide

(WHO 2020a). Among young people aged 12–25 years, depression is the most common mental health problem. In older adults, symptoms of depression can often be misinterpreted as a sign of age-related issues thus misdiagnosis and lack of appropriate treatment can occur. Mood disorders are generally reported by females more than males. In Australia it is estimated that approximately 9.1% of males and 11.6% of females have depression (ABS 2018). Bipolar disorder, on the other hand, develops equally in men and women though the presentation of symptoms and onset may differ. Globally, bipolar disorder affects between 2% and 3% of a population.

Major depressive disorder

Symptoms of major depressive disorder include:

- depressed mood (has to be present for diagnosis)
- loss of pleasure in activities that were previously pleasurable (has to be present for diagnosis)
- significant change in weight (up or down)
- sleep disturbances
- psychomotor agitation or retardation
- loss of energy, or fatigue
- feelings of worthlessness
- impaired concentration
- suicidal ideation.

Bipolar disorder

Bipolar disorder is characterised by episodes of depression (low mood) and mania (heightened mood). These episodes must last at least one week. Manic episodes are characterised by insomnia, boundless energy, inability to concentrate, persistently elevated mood, irritability and fluctuating mood. Depressive episodes have the same criteria as for major depressive disorder. Psychosis can occur when a person experiences extreme mood swings, particularly delusional thinking.

Types of bipolar disorder

Bipolar illness is usually grouped into two types: bipolar I and bipolar II. Although bipolar I is the most studied of the two types, guidance on managing bipolar II is based on data from those studies.

People with bipolar I experience at least one lifetime episode of mania and usually episodes of depression. People with bipolar II experience episodes of depression plus episodes of a mild form of mania called hypomania (persistent elevation of mood, energy and activity). It can take up to 10 years for a diagnosis of this disorder to be made (American Psychiatric Association 2013).

Childbirth and mood disorders

Although childbirth is usually seen as a happy event, some women (up to 50%) and a few men experience postpartum (after birth) 'blues'. Symptoms include anxiety and tearfulness and may be episodic, with the person feeling happy one minute and very upset the next. The cause is unclear, but exhaustion, hormonal changes and stress appear to play a part. If symptoms persist beyond two weeks, medical assessment for postnatal depression is required.

Pre- and postpartum depression

The signs of pre- and postpartum depression are similar to general depression. Postpartum depression (also known as postnatal depression) can develop several months after giving birth. The main symptoms are low mood, poor appetite, altered sleep pattern and low self-esteem. Treatment may involve medication, psychological input and, in some severe cases, electroconvulsive treatment to bring about rapid clinical improvement to allow bonding between mother and baby.

Postpartum psychosis, also referred to as puerperal psychosis, is rare, and it involves a rapid onset, often within 48 hours of giving birth. This condition is characterised by mood swings and psychotic features such as delusions and hallucinations.

Early detection of antenatal and postnatal depression is vital therefore lots of initiatives have been developed to provide better support and treatment for expectant and new mothers experiencing depression.

Treatment

Treatment of mood disorders includes medication to stabilise, raise or lower mood (in mania) and a range of psychotherapies including behaviour therapy and cognitive behaviour therapy. For a small group of people Electroconvulsive therapy (ECT) may be considered. This is most commonly used for those who experience a severe form of depression or severe manic symptoms, or do not improve with medication or other treatments. Occasionally ECT will be used for people who pose a significant and immediate threat to themselves or others since it works quickly in comparison to waiting for other treatments to take effect.

DISORDERS IN YOUNG PEOPLE

There are a range of common mental health conditions experienced by children and young people in the same way as adults. Changes in mood, behaviour, development and learning which cause distress and impact on a child or young person's day-to-day living may mean that help and support is required.

How common?

Attention deficit disorder, anxiety and depression are the most diagnosed mental health issues seen in children, with behavioural problems being frequently diagnosed in younger children (6–11 years) compared with depression and anxiety diagnosed in later years. The World Health Organization estimates 10–20% of children and young people experience mental health problems, with boys affected more than girls, and half of all mental health issues having onset before the age of 14 years (WHO 2020b). Below are a few of the mental health problems that can affect children and young people.

Neurodevelopmental disorders

Neurodevelopmental disorders usually occur early in childhood as a result of impaired brain development contributing to developmental deficits in one or more of areas of functioning, such as socialisation, personal independence, learning and acquisition of skills. This can include autism spectrum disorders, specific learning disorders, global developmental delay and communication disorders. Attention deficit hyperactivity disorder (ADHD) also falls within this range of conditions.

Attention Deficit with Hyperactivity Disorder

ADHD is a neurodevelopmental disorder that is thought to be a syndrome of behaviours where children have more difficulty with concentrating on what they are doing (problems with attention) than other children of their age. Boys are more likely to be diagnosed with this disorder than girls are. Behaviours include:

- lack of attention to detail with schoolwork or other activities
- trouble organising and sticking to tasks and activities
- not following through on instructions (that they are able to understand) and not finishing tasks (e.g. at school or chores at home)
- being easily distracted and forgetful generally
- hyperactivity/impulsivity.

Treatment

Treatment for ADHD is complex but usually involves a multi-modal approach incorporating medication, education, behaviour modification, social skills training and family counselling.

Autism

Autism is a condition that affects how a person communicates with, and relates to, other people. It also affects how they make sense of the world around them.

Core features include:

- persistent difficulties with social communication and social interaction—for example, they may find it hard to begin or carry on a conversation and do not understand social rules such as how far to stand from somebody else
- repetitive patterns of behaviour and interests—for example, they may be very inflexible in their routines or rituals, make repetitive body movements or be very sensitive to certain sounds.

Treatment

Treatment for autism spectrum disorder includes early intensive behavioural interventions with specialised health professionals. Treatment is intensive, time-consuming and very expensive.

INTELLECTUAL DISABILITY

About 1% of the population has an intellectual disability. Intellectual disability is not a mental illness per se; rather it is a neurodevelopment disorder. Reasons for disability vary but include infections, trauma, toxins, problems during childbirth and genetic problems (e.g. Down syndrome, Angelman's syndrome).

Criteria for diagnosis

In the new *DSM-5* less emphasis is placed on an IQ (measure of intelligence) of less than 70 for diagnosis. Instead, it focuses on problems with communication with others and activities of daily living, and lack of independence.

Treatment

Recovery-based models of care focus on personal strengths and maximum level of functioning in the community.

EATING DISORDERS
How common?

Anorexia nervosa is an eating disorder that affects 0.3–0.5% of the population. It affects more females than males (ratio 10:1). Bulimia affects 1–3% of young adult females and is less common in males. Onset usually occurs in late adolescence, and it is more common in Westernised countries.

Anorexia nervosa

There are two main types of anorexia:

- the *restricting type*, where the person inhibits food overall, is less impulsive and there are fewer self-harming behaviours and suicide attempts
- the *bingeing/purging type*, which is characterised by:
  - a family history of obesity or being overweight prior to the condition developing
  - use of vomiting and medications to decrease weight
  - self-harm and suicidal behaviours.

Symptoms

Symptoms include:

- persistent restriction of energy intake leading to significantly low bodyweight (in the context of what is minimally expected for the person's age, sex, developmental trajectory and physical health)
- either an intense fear of gaining weight or of becoming fat or persistent behaviour that interferes with weight gain (even though the person has significantly low weight)
- disturbance in the way the person's bodyweight or shape is experienced, undue influence of body shape and weight on self-evaluation, or persistent lack of recognition of the seriousness of the current low bodyweight (Eating Disorders Victoria 2020).

Physical symptoms of anorexia nervosa include:

- anaemia (low iron blood count)
- bradycardia (low pulse rate)
- eroded teeth enamel
- fine, downy body hair
- hypotension (low blood pressure)
- loss of muscle mass.

Mental health symptoms include:

- depression
- insomnia
- lack of energy
- loss of appetite
- low self-esteem
- obsessive behaviour around food
- poor concentration

- poor memory
- social withdrawal.

Bulimia nervosa

Bulimia nervosa is an eating disorder where the person has patterns of bingeing and purging, causing emotional distress, preoccupation with body shape and weight. The person's bodyweight is often normal.

Behaviours

Behaviours include:

- craving for food
- preoccupation with eating
- a pattern of overeating followed by compensatory behaviour to reverse food intake (exercise or self-induced vomiting).

Physical and psychological symptoms

Symptoms are similar to that for anorexia nervosa, but bodyweight may be within the normal range. Purging-related symptoms include:

- constipation
- electrolyte (salt) imbalance
- irregular heartbeat
- oesophageal/gastric perforation
- stomach ulcers
- tooth decay.

Treatment

Treatment for an eating disorder is dependent on the severity of the condition and can include intensive medical treatment, psychotherapies including cognitive behaviour therapy and family therapy, antidepressant medication and nutritional educational and support.

PERSONALITY DISORDERS

Personality can be defined as a person's lifelong, persistent and enduring characteristics and attitudes, including their ways of thinking, feeling and behaving. These characteristics affect all aspects of a person's life including their work, social and personal relationships. Personality disorders can be defined as abnormal, extreme, inflexible and pervasive variations from the normal range of one or more personality attributes, causing suffering to the person as well as to those around them. Personality has generally formed by about 16 years of age, and so after this age a disorder can be diagnosed. Personality traits are continuous and need to be distinguished from episodic symptoms and behaviours that occur with mental illness.

How common?
About 3% of the general population has a borderline personality disorder—the most common disorder of personality. Rates for other personality disorders are much smaller and hard to establish.

Diagnosing and treating personality disorders remains controversial and problematic because critics of these diagnoses believe that personality, by definition, cannot be changed and is therefore untreatable by the mental health system. Even among health professionals, people with personality disorders are often misunderstood. A common belief is that any exhibited behaviour is within a person's control, i.e. manipulative or used as strategy to gain attention. Responses such as this perpetuate the negative, discriminatory and stigmatising attitudes of health professionals leading to a stereotype of people living with personality disorder and barriers to care. Contemporary research, however, has found links to early childhood trauma (e.g. abuse, abandonment, violence) and emotional dysregulation, similar to that seen in post-traumatic stress disorder. Such understandings enable professionals to see the symptoms of personality disorder as a complex reaction to trauma and work with individuals in context of their history, trauma, and social situation. Health professionals have a responsibility to think about the underlying cause of behaviour and work with people to reduce the distress and suffering they endure on a daily basis due to living with a personality disorder.

Personality disorder group
There are three groups of personality disorders (see Table 4.2).

- *Cluster A.* As a group, these people tend to be perceived as odd, eccentric and withdrawn. This group of personality disorders includes paranoid personality disorder, schizoid personality disorder and schizotypal personality disorder.
- *Cluster B.* People with these disorders appear dramatic, emotional and erratic. This group of personality disorders includes histrionic personality disorder, antisocial personality disorder, narcissistic personality disorder and borderline personality disorder. People with a severe borderline personality disorder or those who have another mental illness such as depression may come into frequent contact with mental health and emergency services when they are in crisis. Careful and consistent management and support is required (see Chapter 7).

TABLE 4.2
Personality disorder groups

Personality disorders by type	Characteristics
Cluster A	
Paranoid	Distrusting and suspicious
	Highly sensitive
Schizoid	Cold and unemotional
	Lack of interest in other people
	Very introspective
Schizotypal	Socially isolative
	Has unusual ideas
	Often has odd behaviours and appearance
Cluster B	
Borderline	Unstable relationships with other people
	Poor self-image
	Unpredictable and erratic moods
	Impulsive substance misuse
	Impulsive self-harming behaviours
Narcissistic	Strong sense of entitlement
	Grandiosity
	Seeks admiration
	Lack of empathy for others
Antisocial	Tendency to violate the boundaries of others
	Superficial charm
	Poor behaviour control: expressions of irritability, threats, aggression and verbal abuse
Histrionic	Excessive attention-seeking behaviours
	Egocentric
	Highly emotional

Continued

TABLE 4.2
Personality disorder groups—cont'd

Personality disorders by type	Characteristics
Cluster C	
Avoidant	Insecure
	Social isolation due to fears of rejection or humiliation by others
Obsessive-compulsive	Preoccupation with orderliness and control over situations
	Rigid behaviour
	Perfectionism
Dependent	Excessive need to be taken care of
	Clinging, submissive
	Feels helpless when not in a relationship

Source: Sadock & Sadock 2007

- *Cluster C.* People with these disorders appear highly anxious and fearful of events and people. This group of personality disorders includes avoidant personality disorder, obsessive-compulsive personality disorder and dependent personality disorder.

Treatment

Treatment for personality disorders focuses on psychotherapeutic approaches—in particular, dialectical behaviour therapy.

DISORDERS IN OLDER PEOPLE
How common?

Delirium is a relatively common health problem in old age, with about 30% of older people admitted to hospital experiencing it. It is marked by an acute disturbance in attention and thinking. Any changes in old age associated with a decline in function or thinking are not normal and need to be investigated and treated.

Delirium is an acute medical condition that can lead to death. It should be treated as a medical emergency. It is not a mental illness or disorder. Rather, it is a reversible clinical syndrome, which is often commonly confused with other disorders such as dementia or depression. Dementia affects about 10% of people aged older than 60 and about 40% of people aged older than 85.

Delirium

Delirium can be precipitated by:

- dehydration or constipation
- drug or alcohol withdrawal
- immobility
- infections
- kidney or liver problems
- lack of sleep
- other disorders (e.g. cancer, neurological disorders)
- pain
- polypharmacy.

The three main criteria for a diagnosis of delirium are:

- attention span impairment
- change in cognitive function or altered perception (e.g. hallucinations, thought disorder)
- rapid onset of symptoms (hours) or fluctuating mental state.

It is extremely important to differentiate between delirium and other disorders such as dementia and depression in order to provide the most appropriate care. Essential differences are listed in Table 4.3.

Memory aid: Depression develops over days and weeks, dementia develops over months and delirium develops over hours.

Dementia

Dementia is a broad term to cover a range of neurocognitive disorders that affects memory, thinking and behaviour. Two main types of dementia are: Alzheimer's disease (more common) and vascular dementia.

Dementia is characterised by one or more of the following cognitive disturbances:

- difficulties with speech
- disturbance of memory
- loss of motor control
- decline from previous level of functioning
- impaired social or occupational abilities and performance.

TABLE 4.3
Differences between delirium, dementia and depression

Mental State Examination	Delirium	Dementia	Depression
Onset	Hours to days	Over months	One or more weeks
Behaviour	Restless and uneasy	Wandering and searching	Slowed, with changes to activities of daily living, eating and sleeping
Cognition	Impaired	Impaired	Slowed, may seem impaired
Attention	Poor/fluctuates	Impaired	May appear impaired
Affect	Changeable; may be irritable or flat, withdrawn	Normal/flat/confused	Sad/irritable/worried/depressed/guilty
Thought	May be incoherent	Shallow; content may be paranoid due to memory problems	Slowed up, guilty thoughts, hypochondria
Judgment	Often impaired	Declining	May seem impaired
Insight	Poor	Reduced	Changeable

Other mental disorders in older people

Older people are particularly prone to depression because of a range of life events including physical illness, isolation, chronic pain and bereavement. Recognising depression in older adults can be difficult as they may show different symptoms than younger adults. They may be more likely to present with recurring physical ailments such as fatigue or pain rather than feelings of sadness in the first instance. Schizophrenia and bipolar disorder are less likely to occur in the older population, but given the chronic nature of these illnesses, older adults may be living with this condition.

Treatment

Treatment for delirium is managed by treating the cause; for example, if the person has a urinary tract infection, antibiotics will be given, or if dehydration is a cause, fluids will be administered. Medication may be required if the person is very distressed or agitated.

Treatment for dementia includes cognitive-enhancing medications, occupational therapy and rehabilitative therapy.

SUBSTANCE RELATED DISORDERS

How common?
The use of alcohol, cannabis, stimulants (amphetamines, cocaine), sedatives (temazepam, oxazepam, diazepam) and opioids (morphine and codeine) is prevalent worldwide. Compared with women, men begin using alcohol and drugs at an earlier age than women; thus, dependence and developing a substance use disorder is twice as likely for males than for females (AIHW 2021). There is a strong link between substance use disorders and other mental health problems particularly underlying anxiety disorder or depression. The use of drugs can trigger or exacerbate a mental health condition. Similarly, many people with a lived experience of mental illness use alcohol and drugs to self-medicate, while not understanding the risk of tolerance and dependency.

Treatment
Treatment for substance-related disorders involves the following steps:

1. Detoxification (the process by which the body rids itself of a drug)
2. Behavioural counselling/motivational counselling
3. Medication (for opioid, tobacco or alcohol addiction)
4. Evaluation and treatment for co-occurring mental health issues such as depression and anxiety.

CONCLUSION
The most common mental illnesses have been included in this chapter as an introduction to the types of symptoms, thoughts, feelings, behaviours and beliefs that people with mental illness may have and suffer from. Groupings of disorders are helpful only in as much as they group symptoms together to gain a clear understanding of what is happening for the person. Some symptoms, such as altered mood, altered perceptions and suicidal feelings, can occur across a range of mental illnesses. Finally, each person with mental illness has a unique experience and, for that reason, carefully designed individualised care by trained health professionals is required.

REFERENCES

American Psychiatric Association. (2013). *Diagnostic and statistical manual of mental disorders (DSM-5)*. Washington DC: American Psychiatric Publishing.

Australian Bureau of Statistics (ABS). (2018). *National health survey: first results – Australia 2017–18*. Canberra: ABS.

Australian Institute of Health & Welfare (AIHW). (2021). *Mental health services in Australia: prevalence, impact and burden*. Online. Available: https://www.aihw. gov.au/reports/mental-health-services/mental-health-services-in-australia/report-contents/summary/prevalence-and-policies 3 March 2021.

Eating Disorders Victoria. (2020). *Classifying eating disorders*. Online. Available: https://www.eatingdisorders.org.au/eating-disorders-a-z/what-is-an-eating-disorder/ 27 February 2021.

Koenen, K.C., Ratanatharathorn, A., Ng, L., et al. (2017). Posttraumatic stress disorder in the World Mental Health Surveys. *Psychological Medicine, 47,* 2260.

Munir, S. & Takov, V. (2020) Generalized Anxiety Disorder. In StatPearls Treasure Island (FL): StatPearls Publishing Online. Available: https://www.ncbi.nlm.nih. gov/books/NBK441870/ 20 February 2020.

Remes, O., Brayne, C., van der Linde, R., & Lafortune, L. (2016). A systematic review of reviews on the prevalence of anxiety disorders in adult populations. *Brain and Behavior, 6*(7), e00497.

Sadock, B. J., & Sadock, V. A. (2007). *Synopsis of psychiatry: behavioral sciences/clinical psychiatry* (10th ed.). Philadelphia: Lippincott Williams.

World Health Organization (WHO). (2017a). Depression and other common mental disorders: global health estimates. Geneva: WHO.

World Health Organization (WHO). (2017b). *International statistical classification of diseases and related health problems, 11th revision (ICD-11)*. Online. Available: http://www.who.int/classifications/icd/en/ 28 April 2017.

World Health Organization (WHO). (2020a). Depression. Geneva: World Health Organization. Online. Available: https://www.who.int/news-room/fact-sheets/detail/depression 27 Feb 2021.

World Health Organization (WHO). (2020b). *Guidelines on mental health promotive and preventive interventions for adolescents: helping adolescents thrive.* Geneva: WHO

WEB RESOURCES

Alzheimer's Australia: www.fightdementia.org.au. This is the peak body providing support and advocacy for the 500,000 Australians living with dementia.

Beyond Blue: www.beyondblue.org.au. Beyond Blue provides information about depression to consumers, carers and health professionals.

Intellectual disability: http://www.intellectualdisability.info/. This is a UK-based information website about the nature of intellectual disability and resources.

Mental Health Foundation of New Zealand: https://www.mentalhealth.org.nz/. A website for consumers and carers to find the latest information on mental health issues.

National Drug Strategy: http://www.nationaldrugstrategy.gov.au. This website provides information about the National Drug Strategy and the advisory structures that support the strategy, links to the current drug campaign sites, key research and data components and links to relevant governments, professional organisations and drug-related portal sites.

National Institute of Mental Health: www.nimh.nih.gov/health/statistics. This website provides data and statistics about mental illnesses in the United States.

Royal College of Psychiatrists UK: www.rcpsych.ac.uk/publications. This website provides information about major mental illnesses for health professionals and the general public.

World Health Organization (WHO): http://www.who.int/topics/mental_disorders/en/. WHO is the health arm of the United Nations and provides up-to-date information on a wide range of health-related data.

5 MENTAL HEALTH ASSESSMENT

INTRODUCTION

This chapter focuses on the essentials of mental health assessment. The purpose, aims and reasons for assessment are described in detail. The mental state examination (MSE), a semi-structured interview that assesses mental functioning, is a crucial component of mental health assessment and is a really useful tool for working with people with a mental health problem. The assessment process is not a tick box checklist but involves developing rapport and engaging with the person you are with. Contemporary mental health assessment also involves identifying the strengths and resources that people have, and their coping skills and abilities, so remember to ask about these also.

WHAT IS A MENTAL HEALTH ASSESSMENT?

Assessment is a method of gathering information in a structured and comprehensive manner. Mental health assessment is a comprehensive, holistic assessment based on the person's developmental, family, social, medical, recreational and employment history. Gently ask about any legal issues such as criminal history as well as recreational drug use. If there is any indication of current suicidal or homicidal ideation, the person must be immediately referred for risk assessment by a qualified mental health clinician.

Mental state assessment includes an MSE and history of current functioning and presenting problems (see Fig. 5.1). The person and family members or carers may contribute perspectives to this assessment. Other standardised assessments (such as specific cognitive or family assessments) may form a part of a comprehensive mental health assessment.

An MSE (also referred to as a 'mental state assessment' (MSA)) is a semi-structured interview to assess another person's current neurological and psychological functioning across several dimensions, such as perception, affect, thought content, form of thought and speech. An MSE

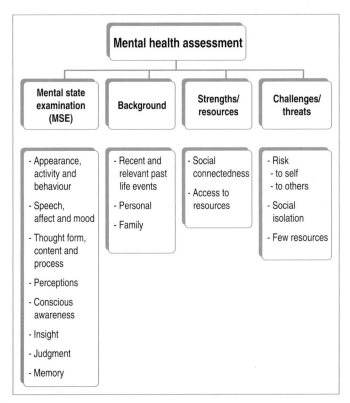

Figure 5.1
Mental health assessment

forms only *part* of an overall mental *health* assessment. For specialised health professionals, including mental health nurses and psychiatrists, the gathering of data for a complete mental health assessment is part of their daily practice and will also identify a person's coping skills, strategies for dealing with stress and supports they can use. For other health workers, such a comprehensive assessment may not be within their scope of practice, and a careful MSE can aid them in providing information to the mental health treating team in order to follow up concerns about a person's mental state.

An MSE can occur at a first meeting as part of a first presentation assessment, during an admission interview, or at any time while communicating with a person. It gathers information about the person's experience and history, with the aim of making informed judgments about the person's need for care and options for care delivery.

An MSE is a 'point in time' assessment and needs to be conducted at regular intervals because a person's mental state may alter or deteriorate rapidly. An initial MSE forms the benchmark for future assessments. Though you may never need to undertake an MSE in its entirety, having a basic understanding enables you to provide accurate information if a referral to mental health services is required. For health professionals such as paramedics, occupational therapists and physiotherapists, the MSE provides a useful snapshot of the person's psychological functioning at the time of the assessment. For people with comorbidities, the MSE allows additional information to be gathered that can inform the necessity for referral to mental health services.

WHY ASSESS?

Reasons for assessment include to:
- engage with the person in a helpful way
- collect information about the person
- allow the person to 'tell their story' (i.e. their understanding of what is happening for them)
- decrease anxiety in the person
- validate that the information they have provided is accurate
- gain a full health picture and make a formulation
- develop an action or treatment plan with the person.

SETTINGS FOR A MENTAL STATE EXAMINATION

The context for assessment will vary according to the setting (e.g. emergency department, community health centre, acute inpatient unit, ambulance call to home, police attendance). Try to find a quiet and safe place to provide privacy, and encourage the person to engage with you. Establishing a relationship with the person is essential in gaining trust and rapport. This may not be possible if you are in a public place. Remember to assess and maintain your own safety before approaching people in distress. Approach slowly but confidently and be careful not to invade their personal space.

CULTURAL ISSUES

It is important to ensure enquiries are made regarding the person's main language spoken and if an interpreter may be required. Religious beliefs may also need to be considered. Factors such as the person's gender and culture and the context in which the assessment is being undertaken need special consideration in order to provide culturally appropriate care.

HOW TO TALK TO FAMILY AND FRIENDS

While your focus is on the person in care, be aware of the need for family and friends to be informed about what is going on. When talking to family and friends:

- offer reassurance and understanding
- listen to their perspective and acknowledge their concerns.

ESSENTIAL MENTAL STATE EXAMINATION SKILLS

Essential skills include the following:

- Ensure your personal safety. Make sure you have a clear exit if in an office space, and don't place yourself in a corner.
- Consider the privacy needs of the person. Some people may prefer to be outside or in an open space, others in a private office.
- *Always* introduce yourself. For example, 'My name is ... and I am a nurse / police officer / ambulance officer / youth worker ...'
- Allow a greater than normal personal space.
- *Listen* carefully.
- Be polite and gentle in your demeanour, but also be clear and direct.
- Observe non-verbal behaviour.
- Be honest in your responses.
- Keep communication open, and allow the person to explain what they think is the current problem.
- Focus your attention on the person (be 'in the moment' with the person).
- Bear in mind that the person may be anxious or fearful.
- Focus on the content of the person's speech, as well as the associated feelings (e.g. sadness, anger) and thoughts (unusual ideas).
- Ask open questions first. Focus on specific, closed questions later on.
- Use paraphrasing to convey to the person that you understand how they are feeling—for example, 'So you say this is the worst you have ever felt? Have I got this right?'
- Don't make promises you cannot keep. For example, don't agree you won't tell anyone else what the person has told you.

Box 5.1 provides tips about taking a good history.

> **Box 5.1   History-taking tips**
>
> - Begin with questions such as 'What has brought you here today?', 'What can I help you with today?' or 'Can you tell me what has been happening for you?'
> - Look like you are listening!
> - Be empathetic and acknowledge how the person is feeling.
> - Repeat the person's statements to seek agreement about what you have heard.
> - Use open and closed questions to gain information.
> - Clarify if needed.
> - Take notes and tell the person why you are writing things down.
> - Show you care by displaying your concern.
> - Make sure you understand the core complaint.
> - If there are multiple concerns ask the person to rank them in order of importance.

THE BASICS AND PURPOSE OF THE MENTAL STATE EXAMINATION

The basics of an MSE are to:

- closely observe and evaluate the person's appearance and behaviour
- listen attentively to the content of speech, which usually reflects thoughts and thinking ability
- ask specific questions about the person's thoughts, feelings and perceptual experiences
- document your assessment and determine a plan of action. Remember that undertaking an MSE is not an end in itself.

Conducting an MSE provides the framework for your plan of care. Its purpose is to:

- clarify the nature of a person's mental health problems
- evaluate a person's present mental state
- identify areas for immediate intervention (e.g. relapse)
- provide a baseline so that a future MSE can evaluate changes in the person's condition and responses to treatment.

THE COMPONENTS OF A MENTAL STATE EXAMINATION

Fig. 5.2 illustrates the eight components of an MSE, beginning with appearance, physical activity and behaviour, then moving to observations that can be made before and during conversing with the person and continuing through to insight and judgment assessments.

1. Appearance, physical activity and behaviour

Appearance

The purpose of this section of the MSE is to describe the general appearance of the person to get a sense of their ability to conduct their personal

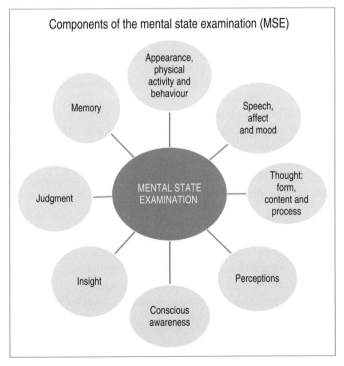

Figure 5.2
Components of a mental state examination

activities of daily living and the appropriateness of their attire. Noting physical characteristics can be useful (e.g. for future identification). The following can be noted:

- gender and ethnicity
- general appearance, chronological age and apparent age
- physical characteristics such as body build, posture and any distinguishing marks
- clothing, including condition of clothes, cleanliness and appropriateness to weather conditions
- grooming, including peculiarities of dress, use of cosmetics, jewellery and hairstyle
- gait (how a person walks).

Physical activity and behaviour

The aim of this section is to describe what the person does in terms of observable behaviour, manner and attitude. Record your observations of:

- posture, gait, gestures, tics, grimaces, tremors and mannerisms
- activity (e.g. overactive or underactive, purposeful or disorganised, pacing, restless, sedentary)[1]
- any signs of physical slowing down
- facial expression (e.g. alert, tense, worried, happy, sad, frightened, angry, laughing, smiling, suspicious)
- rapport with the interviewer (friendly, aloof)
- attitude during the interview (e.g. indifferent, friendly, dramatic, evasive, sullen, irritable, afraid, impulsive, embarrassed, sexually provocative).

2. Speech, affect and mood

This section includes how the person talks (e.g. quantity, rate, volume). Use the following prompts as a guide:

- Is the person's speech soft, loud, stuttering or hesitant?
- Is the flow of speech even or uneven, slow or rapid?
- Does the person's speech contain references to disordered, negative, unrealistic or unusual thoughts?

---

[1] 'Avolition' refers to having a distinct lack of motivation and energy to undertake activities.

Affect

Affect refers to the feeling or emotional state inferred by the assessor on the basis of the person's statements, appearance and behaviour at the time of the assessment. Affect involves observable behaviours such as hand and body movements, facial movements and the tone and pitch of a person's voice. Table 5.1 lists a range of descriptors for affect. Other descriptors include aloof, apathetic, complacent, composed, dull, elated, grandiose, tense, worried and euthymic (normal mood).

Mood

Mood refers to the person's subjective statement about their emotional state—their own description of their internal feeling or emotion—over the past few days and is pervasive and sustained over that time. Mood might be either:

- depressed, happy or sad
- neutral or apathetic[2]
- irritable, anxious or angry
- fearful or euphoric.

TABLE 5.1
Descriptors for affect

Affect	Descriptor
Full range	What would normally be expected in variations of facial expression and gestures
Blunted	Reduction in the emotions expressed or low intensity
Flat	Absence of expressed emotion. Voice might be monotonous and face immobile
Inappropriate or incongruent	Outward expression of the emotional state is not congruent with what the person is expressing
Labile	Expressed emotion fluctuates or is variable beyond normal expression. A person is tearful one minute then angry the next
Restricted	Limited variability of expressed emotion

---

[2]The term 'anhedonia' refers to the person not being able to experience any pleasure in aspects of daily life.

3. Thought: form, content and process

Thought form

Form refers to the amount of thought and its rate of production, such as:

- lack of ideas (cannot identify any thoughts)
- flight of ideas (cannot remain on one topic)
- loose associations (thinking jumps around without apparent connection)
- slow or hesitant.

The assessor makes an assessment of the person's thoughts. Are they able to communicate normally? Do their thoughts appear to be logical and organised? Provide examples to illustrate your assessment.

Thought content

Content refers to the topics or areas that one thinks about. Assessment involves making a judgment about what the person is saying. Does it make sense? Are the ideas related and do they flow logically from one to the next? For example, is the person experiencing any delusional thinking? Is the person ruminating about particular ideas? It is important to ask the person if they have suicidal, self-harm or homicidal thoughts. Sensitivity is required, and follow-up questions are important. Be aware that some people have fleeting or occasional thoughts of suicide for many years but do not act on them.

Delusions

Delusions are known as fixed false beliefs or uncompromising beliefs held in the face of incontrovertible evidence to the contrary and that are not consistent with one's cultural or religious beliefs. Examples of delusions are:

- *Persecutory delusions.* The person has thoughts that life events are in the form of punishment for past wrongdoings.
- *Grandiose delusions.* The person believes they possess unusual talents, virtue, insight or identity.
- *Delusions of reference.* The person believes ordinary events have special meaning or significance only intended for themselves.
- *Delusions of influence.* The person believes others are controlling or manipulating them.
- *Religious delusions.* The person believes they have a special link with a deity. Delusions can also involve the following:
- *Thought insertion.* The person believes others are putting thoughts into their head.
- *Thought broadcasting.* The person believes others can hear or know what they are thinking.
- *Thought withdrawal.* The person believes someone is taking away their thoughts.

Obsessions

Obsessions are involuntary and unwelcome ideas that intrude on the person's other thoughts that then demand their attention, even though the person may recognise them as irrational (e.g. a fear of being contaminated when touching door handles or other surfaces).

Compulsions

Compulsions are insistent, repetitive and unwanted urges to perform a certain act (e.g. wash their hands 10 or more times after going to the toilet).

Thought process

Thought process refers to the movement and dynamics of how one thought connects to the next. Thought process may be any of the following.

- *Logical thought.* Analyses are well-founded and make sense.
- *Loose associations.* Thinking is disorganised and jumps from one idea to another with little apparent connection. *Flight of ideas* is also relevant here where the person cannot remain on one topic.
- *Word salad.* Real words and sometimes neologisms are used, but there is no connection between the words that convey any sense of meaning to the listener.
- *Echolalia.* The person repeats what is said to them.
- *Clang association.* One word follows the next based on similarity of sound or rhyming.
- *Perseveration.* The person continues to repeat an idea, phrase or word, and has trouble shifting to a new thought or idea.

4. Perceptions

Perceptions refer to the person's experience of their world through their senses (their interpretation). The following experiences are false or misperceptions usually associated with mental illness.

Hallucinations

A hallucination is a false sensory perception that occurs without an actual external stimulus. Hallucinations can involve all five senses:

- *Auditory.* These are the most common type of hallucination and often involve voices but can also be humming, tapping, music or laughing.
- *Visual.* These are common in mental disorders with a physical cause (e.g. substance abuse) and involve seeing objects, people or images that others are not able to see.
- *Olfactory.* These are common in mental disorders with a physical cause and involve smelling things that do not exist (e.g. gas from the gas fire

or oven, but it is important to check that the gas has not in fact been left on).

- *Gustatory.* These are most common in organic mental disorders and involve a sense of an unexplained taste in the mouth.
- *Tactile.* These are commonly experienced during a delirium and involve a false perception of touch or sensation (e.g. insects crawling on or under the skin).

Illusions
An illusion is a misinterpretation of an actual external stimulus (e.g. seeing a coat hanging on the wall and thinking that it is a person standing in the room).

Depersonalisation
Depersonalisation refers to a feeling of unreality where the perception of self seems different or unfamiliar (e.g. a person may describe a sense of not being a part of their body or having an out-of-body experience). This sensation is often associated with stress, fatigue and extreme anxiety.

Derealisation
Derealisation refers to the sense that the external world feels unreal, different or altered. People report feeling distanced or cut off from the world. This experience is also associated with stress, fatigue and extreme anxiety.

5. Conscious awareness

Level of consciousness
Level of consciousness refers to the overall state of alertness and may be any of the following:

- *Alert.* The person is awake, fully aware and responsive.
- *Lethargic.* The person is drowsy but responds when spoken to. They may fall asleep.
- *Stuperous.* The person is difficult to rouse, may groan or may become restless when attempts are made to rouse them.
- *Coma.* The person is unresponsive to voice or painful stimuli.

Orientation
This includes orientation to:

- *time*—orientation to hour, day, month and year
- *place*—this relates to whether the person can identify which hospital, city and country they are in
- *person*—this relates to orientation to self or others.

Concentration

Concentration is usually assessed by asking the person to count back from 100 in serial sevens (ask the person to take seven from 100, seven from 93, etc.), spell 'world' backwards or repeat a three-part task.

Abstract thinking

Abstract thinking refers to the ability to deal with concepts and to extract meaning, to understand the meaning of phrases beyond their literal interpretation or to juggle more than one idea at a time. Asking the person to explain the meaning of a common proverb is a good way for some people to assess abstract thinking ability. Examples are:

- All that glitters is not gold.
- When the cat's away the mice will play.
- Don't count your chickens before they hatch.
- Rome wasn't built in a day.

However, understanding of the above proverbs presumes a level of educational attainment (about eight years) and assumes an understanding of Western culture, so proverbs will not be a useful tool with all people. The assessor needs to explain what a proverb is (a saying that has a broader meaning) and provide an example before assessing the person. You can assess higher intellectual functions like abstraction in other ways such as asking, 'How are an apple and an orange both alike?' The expected abstract answer would be 'fruit' and a concrete answer (showing less intellectual function) would be 'that they are both round'. Concrete answers often signal a deficit in intellectual functioning and require further investigation.

6. Insight

Insight is the degree to which the person realises the significance of their symptoms or illness and their current situation, or the degree of self-understanding. Consider the following:

- Is there an appreciation of how their illness may affect their life?
- Do they think they have an illness?
- Do they have full or partial understanding of their situation?
- Are they able to explain why an ambulance has been called?

7. Judgment

Judgment is the ability to make sensible decisions based on expected consequences in everyday activities and social situations. Consider the following:

- Are judgments socially appropriate?

- Are judgments about personal relationships appropriate?
- Is the person able to manage his or her own finances?

Be aware that the concepts of insight and judgment are increasingly being challenged regarding their usefulness in assessing a person's mental health because they are recognised as subjective, contested and loaded concepts.

8. Memory

Memory includes:

- *Remote past recall.* This is the ability of the person to present a coherent life story with dates and places (e.g. birth, employment, relationships).
- *Recent past recall.* This is the ability of the person to recall the history and events leading to their hospitalisation.
- *Immediate past recall.* This is the ability of the person to recall a person's name and three unrelated facts five minutes after being given them.

SUMMARY

An MSE should include a summary statement containing a formulation of what the central issues are and the reasons for admission, and a brief problem list. For further detail, see Evans and colleagues (2017).

CASE STUDY

A Mental State Examination

Phillipa is a single 31-year-old female with previous admissions to a mental health facility for acute psychosis. She has been given a diagnosis of schizophrenia. Phillipa has called an ambulance at 7.30 pm because she is convinced there is a man outside her house who is spying on her. She asks the ambulance staff to find the man and call the police to take him away.

Appearance, physical activity and behaviour

Phillipa answers the door in her pyjamas and a dressing gown. Her hair is not brushed, but she appears clean and appropriately dressed for a cool autumn evening. Her height is about 162 cm, and she has a slim build.

She exhibits a closed posture, sitting hunched up on her lounge, rocking slightly and chewing skin around her fingernails. There is occasional appropriate but brief eye contact. She appears tense and anxious. The living room is clean but untidy. There are few furnishings and the curtains are drawn (but it is dark outside). She admits to keeping the curtains drawn during the day.

Speech, affect and mood

Phillipa is softly spoken, and her speech exhibits normal rate and flow. Her main concern is that a man is waiting outside, and she thinks he is going to break in and hurt her. Because of this, she is sleeping poorly and refuses to leave the house.

She exhibits labile affect and pervasive anxiety. She is suspicious of ambulance staff and tearful at times. She is responding minimally to verbal reassurance.

Thought: form, content and process

Thought form appears normal. For thought content, there is a preoccupation with the man who she thinks is outside her house. She has been outside to check but thinks he hides when she ventures out.

Perceptions

Phillipa describes feeling outside her body (depersonalisation) and being cut off from the world (derealisation).

Conscious awareness

Phillipa is alert and oriented to time, place and person. Her memory is fully intact. Her concentration is poor and she is easily distracted (e.g. by street noise).

Insight

Phillipa does not relate her belief of being watched by a stranger to her mental illness.

Judgment

Phillipa's judgment is impaired due to her mental state. She is unwilling to leave her house and is unable to plan her day because she is persistently worried about being harmed.

ADDITIONAL INFORMATION REQUIRED FOR A MENTAL HEALTH ASSESSMENT
Presenting information

For the overall mental health assessment, a statement is required of the actual reason for the presentation, the nature of the presenting problem and the history of the presenting problem, including precipitating factors and recent stressors. In particular:

- note the history of concordance with the current treatment regimen if any
- identify if there are any urgent social issues that may need to be addressed
- provide a brief outline of the support structures available to the person
- identify the person's strengths and any predisposing, precipitating and perpetuating factors.

Medical history

Medical history includes:

- previous operations, illnesses and admissions to hospital
- family history of illness, medications and allergies
- drug and alcohol use
- nutritional state (weight gain/loss), energy levels, sleep/rest patterns and exercise levels.

Psychiatric history

This section includes a brief summary of:

- any episodes of illness, including admissions to inpatient units, and types of treatments/interventions that were helpful or unhelpful
- attitude to mental health services and treatment
- premorbid personality and level of functioning
- family history
- current mental health services involved in care.

Risk assessment

The mental health assessment should contain a risk assessment, including risk of harm to self or others, risk of abuse by family members (elder abuse and domestic violence), risk of falls and risk of poor nutrition.

Social history

Social history includes:

- developmental history (childhood illnesses, life events, education)
- current family structure (marital status, dependants, significant relationships)
- housing situation
- social supports, employment and occupational history

- financial situation
- forensic history/legal issues
- spiritual and cultural considerations.

It is important to identify a person's personal strengths and resources as well as challenges in order to gain a holistic person-centred assessment.

Drug and alcohol screening

With the increasing evidence of co-occurring mental health problems and alcohol and drug use, it is worthwhile to assess a person's risk of alcohol and drug use to establish if their substance use is problematic and associated with the current mental state. Assessing a person's frequency, level and risk provides an initial brief measure to provide information as to whether a further detailed assessment and treatment is required.

Physical assessment

Having a mental illness is associated with higher rates of complex medical comorbidity and so within any mental health assessment, there should also be screening for acute physical conditions, or ongoing chronic physical health issues. Most emergency departments are required to medically clear anyone presenting with acute disturbance that could possibly be a mental health issue before being referred for evaluation from the specialist mental health team. Unfortunately, in some cases, due to complex presentations, poor communication and time pressures in a busy environment, there is disparity in the physical health assessment and care people with a mental illness receive, whereby health providers focus on the mental state more so than the physical health state. This is called 'diagnostic overshadowing'.

CONCLUSION

This chapter has provided the essential elements of a mental health assessment. Careful gathering of information and engagement with the person will allow useful care to be planned in partnership. It is important to practise assessment skills to become proficient in this activity.

REFERENCE

Evans, K., Nizette, D., & O'Brien, A. (2017). *Psychiatric and mental health nursing* (4th ed.). Sydney: Elsevier.

RESOURCES

The SAD PERSONS mnemonic (Sex, Age, Depression, Prior suicidality/self-harm, Ethanol: alcohol misuse, Rational thinking, Support systems, Organised support system, No significant other, Sickness is a quick easy assessment of suicidality and risk. It is *not* a rating instrument, just a jog for the memory and has no validity in predicting future self-harm.

The Annual Population Survey (UK) includes four questions used to monitor wellbeing. These are:

1. Overall, how satisfied are you with your life nowadays?
2. Overall, to what extent do you feel the things you do in your life are worthwhile?
3. Overall, how happy did you feel yesterday?
4. Overall, how anxious did you feel yesterday?

These are not diagnostic but can be used by health professionals to start a meaningful conversation about how people are feeling generally.

ASSESSMENT SCALES

AUDIT (Alcohol Users Disorders Identification Test) alcohol assessment scale: www.therightmix.gov.au. AUDIT detects excessive and harmful patterns of alcohol and is quick to complete and simple to score.

CAGE (Cut down, Annoyed, Guilty, Eye opener) alcohol screening test: https://www.healthline.com/health/cage-questionnaire. This one of the oldest and most popular screening tools for alcohol misuse. It is a short, four-question test that diagnoses alcohol problems over a lifetime.

Impact of Events Scale: https://www.healthfocuspsychology.com.au/tools/ies-r/. This is a scale of current subjective distress related to a specific event and is based on a list of items composed of commonly reported experiences of intrusion and avoidance.

Kessler Psychological Distress Scale (K10) Anxiety and depression checklist: https://www.worksafe.qld.gov.au/__data/assets/pdf_file/0010/22240/kessler-psychological-distress-scale-k101.pdf. This 10-item questionnaire provides an overall measure of distress based on questions about anxiety and depressive symptoms that a person has experienced in the preceding four weeks.

Mini Psychiatric Assessment Schedule for Adults with Developmental Disabilities (Mini PAS-ADD): www.pasadd.co.uk. This is an accessible assessment tool based on a life-events checklist and the person's symptoms.

Mini-Mental State Examination (MMSE): https://www.ihpa.gov.au/sites/default/files/publications/smmse-tool-v2.pdf. This is an abbreviated form of the mental state examination (MSE) based on observable behaviour in an assessment interview.

Minnesota Multiphasic Personality Inventory: https://psychcentral.com/lib/minnesota-multiphasic-personality-inventory-mmpi. This is a common personality test used by mental health professionals to examine personality structure and psychopathology.

Positive and Negative Symptoms Scale (PANSS): https://www.psychdb.com/_media/psychosis/panss.pdf. PANSS is a medical scale used for measuring symptom severity in patients with schizophrenia.

Rowland Universal Dementia Assessment Scale (RUDAS): https://www.dementia.org.au/resources/rowland-universal-dementia-assessment-scale-rudas. This is a short multicultural cognitive assessment scale.

WEB RESOURCES

Palmerston Association Inc.: https://tnicholson2013.files.wordpress.com/2014/01/msedvdbookletoct2011highresolution.pdf. *Understanding the Mental State Examination (MSE): A basic training guide* is funded by the Australian Government under the Improved Services for People with Drug and Alcohol Problems and Mental Illness through the Department of Health.

University of Bristol: http://www.bristol.ac.uk/medical-school/hippocrates/psychiatry/mse_etc/. This website contains teaching resources developed by the University of Bristol for their undergraduate medical students and offers valuable information on mental health assessment.

6 ASSESSING RISK

INTRODUCTION

This chapter introduces the concept of risk assessment and specifically the importance of mental health risk assessment. 'Risk assessment' refers to the role of the health professional assessing possible risk to the overall health and safety of a person and those around them. Risk assessment is important so that health professionals can decide on an appropriate plan of action with, and for, the person to reduce the likelihood of an adverse event occurring. In mental health, risk assessment often requires appraisal in a wider holistic context thus a biopsychosocial assessment considering the person's psychological wellbeing, physical health and social factors is taken into account. The health professional needs to establish a therapeutic working relationship with the person and assess their needs, with a focus (where possible) on strengths, coping strategies and social supports. The information in this chapter will be useful to see how risk assessment leads onto 'risk management' wherein a plan of care is designed to address identified needs and to continue to assess and evaluate the efficacy of planned interventions.

WHY ASSESS RISK?

Risk assessment does not replace care planning. It is a useful aspect of the overall process of care planning. Risk assessment ought to be done *with* the person; it is not something that is done *to* the person. The core issue with risk assessment is to establish the level of risk (low, medium or high) so that plans can be made to protect the person (i.e. keep them safe) and others. Further, establishing what strengths and resilience the person has can reduce risks and give the person confidence that they have some control in their lives. Questions to ask are highlighted in Box 6.1.

Risk assessment is *not* about making predictions about certain events and is only an assessment of the current situation. Remember that when

---

Box 6.1 Risk assessment questions

- What is the risk?
- Who is at risk?
- What is the chance of the risk occurring?
- How immediate is the risk?
- Over what timeframe is the risk being assessed?
- What factors can increase or decrease the risk (e.g. stressors, people, situations)?
- Are alcohol or other drugs involved?
- What do we need to do to reduce or manage the risk?
- What is the plan of action?

---

asking people about their suicidal intent, for example, your assessment relies on what they tell you, which you have to accept as true. While health professionals cannot in any certainty predict if a person will have an outcome that is fatal for themselves or another person, they can perform a risk assessment to identify potential risk factors that support clinical practice in response to what has been heard.

Risk in mental health contexts generally refers to acute immediate risk issues, such as the risk of harm to self or others, but it can take many forms. It includes the risk of:

- absconding (leaving hospital without permission)
- adverse effects of medication (e.g. side effects, toxicity)
- danger to self and others
- falls
- financial, physical or sexual exploitation
- gambling
- harassment or stalking
- homelessness
- not taking psychiatric medication
- notoriety due to bizarre behaviour
- obesity and other illness
- physical health deterioration
- poverty or self-neglect

- reckless behaviour such as unsafe driving
- sexual promiscuity
- social isolation
- substance abuse
- unemployment
- verbal or physical abuse.

It is important for health professionals to be aware of the less obvious but significant risks that people with a mental illness face and the effect that these risks can have on their day-to-day functioning. Being homeless and socially isolated, or being dependent on drugs or alcohol, increases day-to-day stresses and can contribute to an increase in self neglect, symptoms of mental illness or distressed behaviour such as self-harming.

Box 6.2 lists the core principles for working with risk.

TYPES OF RISK FACTOR

Some risk factors are termed **static** because they are fixed, such as gender or history of violence. They cannot be changed and give a baseline of how someone might behave. **Dynamic** risk factors are factors that can change in duration and intensity, such as hopelessness, agitation and substance abuse. These can be measured, and it is important to try and minimise the distress such factors can cause so that people have the opportunity to progress in their recovery and mental wellbeing.

For a few people, experiencing an acutely distressed state of mental health can impact on their behaviour and cause concern associated with

---

Box 6.2   Core principles for working with risk

- Risk is a normal part of life.
- Risk can be minimised but not eliminated.
- Risk changes with time and circumstances.
- Identifying a risk carries a duty to do something about it (risk management plan).
- The person's own involvement is vital.
- Risk assessment requires multiple sources of information including from the person, carers and clinicians.

Source: Morgan 2004

> **Box 6.3** Risk factors in aggression/violence
>
> - Being male, under 35 years of age
> - Having psychosis, dementia, organic brain injury, personality disorder
> - History of substance misuse (alcohol or drugs)
> - Recent life stressors
> - Previous history of violence
> - History of prison incarceration
> - Unstable living arrangements
> - Disengagement from mental health services
>
> Source: Adapted from Hart 2014

elevated risk. Two such areas are violence (see Box 6.3) and suicide (Box 6.4), therefore it is important to be able to recognise and identify the risk factors for each. Suicidal intent is often associated with mental illness (WHO, 2019), however there are a number of deaths by suicide that are not attributable to mental illness. Similarly, the same could be argued for aggressive and violent behaviour. Although there is evidence linking severe mental illness and violent behaviour, this accounts for a small percentage with most people presenting no increased risk (Silverstein et al 2015).

WHEN TO DO RISK ASSESSMENT

Risk assessment is vital when first meeting a person or when there is a transfer of care, change in clinical condition or deterioration in mental state. The most reliable person regarding a risk assessment is the last person who made the assessment. In a crisis situation a comprehensive risk assessment is not immediately required; undertake an immediate high-risk assessment and formulate a plan of care.

WHAT IS IN A MENTAL HEALTH RISK ASSESSMENT?

Mental health risk assessment involves collecting relevant background information, using the risk assessment your organisation prefers, structuring an individual assessment to predict risk and formulating a risk management plan.

There are a number of tools to assess risk in clinical settings usually involving checklists or scales that predict a low-, medium- or high-risk outcome of harm occurring. These are generally about risk of violence

Box 6.4	Risk factors for suicide

- Being single
- Being unemployed
- Being divorced or widowed
- Being male, younger than 25 or older than 85 years of age
- Being of Indigenous heritage
- Recent life stressors
- History of prison incarceration
- Having a mental illness
- Discharge from a psychiatric inpatient unit within 14 days
- History of substance misuse (alcohol or drugs)
- Expressing excessive guilt
- Poor physical health
- Social isolation
- Expressing hopelessness or helplessness

or suicide. They can be a useful adjunct to the risk assessment interview. Remember though that the use of a rating scale is not a risk assessment in itself, it is merely a prompt as part of the wider risk assessment process. Clinical judgment, building a rapport and collecting quality information in context of a person's age, developmental issues, gender, culture, strengths and resources, and shared decision making including family and carers when possible, supports a quality and effective mental health risk assessment process.

WHAT TO TELL THE PERSON WHEN UNDERTAKING A RISK ASSESSMENT

The person needs to be informed at the beginning of the interaction:

- how long the assessment will take or how much time you have available
- that some questions may be uncomfortable to answer but are important in order to provide good care
- that the person can refuse to answer questions, but the more information gained, the better the care that can be provided
- what happens next. (Hart 2014)

MAKING A FORMULATION AND MANAGEMENT PLAN

The risk formulation summarises the information gathered in the assessment and identifies the risks. It usually contains the following elements.

- Background: demographics, culture, history of harm to self or others
- Current situation: stressors, precipitating events
- Risk factors: what they are and what priority they are
- Risk status: low-, medium- and high-risk level assessed
- Timeframe: when the next assessment is due.

The management plan is an important part of the process. It aims to set out what specifically should happen to manage the risk identified, future preventive actions, protective factors the person has to employ, the plan for likely future risk and what the person can do in a crisis. It is the next step whereby responsibilities of those involved are identified and converted into tangible actions often developed as part of a care plan. A risk management plan will have clear review dates.

An example of a risk assessment and management template can be found on the following pages.

MENTAL HEALTH RISK ASSESSMENT AND MANAGEMENT TEMPLATE

General risk factors	
Background factors	
Major psychiatric illness	☐Y ☐N ☐Unknown
Diagnosed personality disorder	☐Y ☐N ☐Unknown
History of substance misuse	☐Y ☐N ☐Unknown
Serious medical condition	☐Y ☐N ☐Unknown
Intellectual disability/cognitive deficits	☐Y ☐N ☐Unknown
Significant behavioural disturbance (< 18 years)	☐Y ☐N ☐Unknown
Childhood abuse/mistreatment	☐Y ☐N ☐Unknown
Current factors	
Disorientation/disorganisation	☐Y ☐N ☐Unknown
Disinhibition/intrusive/impulsive behaviour	☐Y ☐N ☐Unknown
Current intoxication/withdrawal	☐Y ☐N ☐Unknown

Continued

Significant physical pain	☐Y ☐N ☐Unknown
Emotional distress/agitation	☐Y ☐N ☐Unknown

Comments:

Suicide risk factors	
Background factors	
Previous suicide attempts	☐Y ☐N ☐Unknown
History of self-harm	☐Y ☐N ☐Unknown
Family history of suicide	☐Y ☐N ☐Unknown
Separated/widowed/divorced	☐Y ☐N ☐Unknown
Isolation or lack of support/supervision	☐Y ☐N ☐Unknown
Current factors	
Recent significant life events	☐Y ☐N ☐Unknown
Hopelessness/despair	☐Y ☐N ☐Unknown
Experiencing high levels of distress	☐Y ☐N ☐Unknown
Expressing suicidal ideas	☐Y ☐N ☐Unknown
Self-harming behaviour	☐Y ☐N ☐Unknown
Current plan/intent	☐Y ☐N ☐Unknown
Access to means	☐Y ☐N ☐Unknown

Comments:

Violence/aggression risk factors	
Background factors	
Previous incidents of violence	☐Y ☐N ☐Unknown
Previous use of weapons	☐Y ☐N ☐Unknown
Forensic history	☐Y ☐N ☐Unknown

Previous dangerous/violent ideation	☐Y ☐N ☐**Unknown**
Current factors	
Recent violence	☐Y ☐N ☐**Unknown**
Command hallucinations	☐Y ☐N ☐**Unknown**
Violence-related restraining order	☐Y ☐N ☐**Unknown**
Paranoid ideation about others	☐Y ☐N ☐**Unknown**
Expressing intent to harm others	☐Y ☐N ☐**Unknown**
Anger/agitation	☐Y ☐N ☐**Unknown**
Poor impulse control	☐Y ☐N ☐**Unknown**
Access to available means	☐Y ☐N ☐**Unknown**
Contact with vulnerable people	☐Y ☐N ☐**Unknown**
Comments:	
Other risk factors	
Background factors	
History of absconding	☐Y ☐N ☐**Unknown**
History of physical/sexual victimisation	☐Y ☐N ☐**Unknown**
History of gambling or poor control of finances	☐Y ☐N ☐**Unknown**
History of falls/accidents	☐Y ☐N ☐**Unknown**
History of exploitation by others	☐Y ☐N ☐**Unknown**
History of neglect of a serious medical condition	☐Y ☐N ☐**Unknown**
History of non-adherence to medication/treatment	☐Y ☐N ☐**Unknown**
Current factors	
Desire to leave hospital	☐Y ☐N ☐**Unknown**
Vulnerability to sexual exploitation/abuse	☐Y ☐N ☐**Unknown**
Current delusional beliefs	☐Y ☐N ☐**Unknown**
Parental/carer status or access to children	☐Y ☐N ☐**Unknown**

Continued

Physical illness	☐Y ☐N ☐Unknown
Self-neglect, poor self-care	☐Y ☐N ☐Unknown
Non-adherence to medications/treatment	☐Y ☐N ☐Unknown
Impaired cognition/judgment	☐Y ☐N ☐Unknown
Impulsive/reckless driving	☐Y ☐N ☐Unknown

Comments:

Protective factors (list)

Identified strengths & resources (list)

Overall impression

Is the person's level of risk highly changeable?	☐Yes ☐No
Are there factors that contribute uncertainty regarding the level of risk?	☐Yes ☐No

Overall assessment of risk

Suicide	☐H ☐M ☐L
Self-harm	☐H ☐M ☐L
Violence/aggression	☐H ☐M ☐L
Vulnerability	☐H ☐M ☐L
Absconding	☐H ☐M ☐L

Other (describe) _____	☐H ☐M ☐L
_____	☐H ☐M ☐L

Specific risks to be addressed in management plan (list)

CASE STUDY

Julie-Anne is a 27-year-old woman with a history of self-harming behaviour (cutting her arms with a razor blade). A member of the public calls an ambulance and police to a car park after seeing Julie-Anne sitting on the ground, drinking from a wine bottle and holding a large kitchen knife. Julie-Anne has slurred speech, and the paramedic notices a bottle of rat poison in a shopping bag by her side. Julie-Anne says her boyfriend has ended their relationship earlier that day and she has nothing left to live for. Table 6.1 shows how you might formulate the risk in this case.

TABLE 6.1
Formulating the risk

Who is at risk?	Julie-Anne, attending paramedics and police
What is the risk?	Risk of self-harm and harm to others
What are the risk factors for Julie-Anne?	Intoxication, recent separation, previous history of self-harm, possession of poison, possession of and holding a large knife, feeling hopeless
What is the level of severity of the risk?	High

REFERENCES

Hart, C. (2014). A pocket guide to risk assessment and management. Oxon, Great Britain: Routledge.

Morgan, S. (2004). Risk taking. In P. Ryan & S. Morgan (Eds.), *Assertive outreach: a strengths based approach to policy and practice.* London: Churchill Livingstone.

Silverstein, S. M., Del Pozzo, J., Roché, M., et al. (2015). Psychosis and violence: realities, recommendations, and implications for offender profiling. *Crime Psychology Review, 1,* 21-42.

World Health Organization (WHO). (2019). Suicide. Geneva: WHO. Online. Available: https://www.who.int/news-room/fact-sheets/detail/suicide 12 May 2021.

WEB RESOURCES

Headspace: Assessing & Responding to Safety Concerns: https://headspace.org.au/clinical-toolkit/assessing-and-responding-to-safety-concerns/. This site offers valuable information when working with children and young people.

Ministry of Health. 2016. *Preventing suicide: guidance for emergency departments.* Wellington: Ministry of Health: https://www.health.govt.nz/publication/preventing-suicide-guidance-emergency-departments. Information about people at risk of suicide in emergency departments developed by Te Pou o te Whakaaro Nui.

NICE: Violence and aggression: short-term management in mental health, health and community settings. NICE guideline NG10; 2015: https://www.nice.org.uk/guidance/ng10/chapter/1-Recommendations#preventing-violence-and-aggression-2. This resource contains recommendations on how to manage violence and aggression in the short term to avoid escalation of a serious incident.

Queensland Health 2019 Violence Risk assessment and management framework – mental health services, State of Queensland: https://www.health.qld.gov.au/__data/assets/pdf_file/0027/856242/viol-risk-framework.pdf. This document offers a framework that supports care for consumers who may pose a risk of violence towards others.

square – suicide, questions, answers and resources: https://www.square.org.au/risk-assessment/risk-assessment-guide/. 'square' is an educational resource for primary healthcare and community specialists and anyone working with people who are at risk of suicide.

The Centre for Best Practice in Aboriginal and Torres Strait Islander Suicide Prevention, Screening and Assessment Tools: https://www.cbpatsisp.com.au/our-research/screening-assessment-tools/. This site offers many resources to promote best practice when working within a cultural context.

7 BEHAVIOURS OF CONCERN

INTRODUCTION

This chapter explores behaviours of concern in the context of people experiencing mental health problems. These behaviours include situations in which a person is in extreme distress (e.g. having a panic attack, being violent, intoxicated or suicidal or having experienced a trauma). In such situations, the role of health professionals is to assess the situation with a primary focus on risk assessment in terms of the person harming themselves or others (i.e. the bottom line is to maintain safety for everyone). A situation where someone is angry or aggressive does not, in itself, constitute an emergency if the person can be helped to calm down. Health professionals may come across a wide range of people whose behaviours challenge them. Such people may already be well known to health professionals, emergency and mental health services and require patience and a willingness to engage with them, considering why such behaviour is being presented. Specific strategies are suggested here.

BEHAVIOURS OF CONCERN

Many people using health and social services exhibit challenging behaviours for a variety of reasons. The behaviour may be problematic for them or for others around them. For any support or help to be effective, it is essential for health professionals to remember it is the behaviour that is a problem and not the person. Frequent examples of behaviours of concern include:

- frequent presentations to emergency departments
- frequent calls to ambulance or police
- frequent non-life-threatening self-harming behaviours
- repeated overdose of prescription or non-prescription medicines
- alcohol and substance intoxication
- aggressive or violent outbursts
- refusing to do things.

It is important to remember that when people are in crisis they may behave in ways that we consider unacceptable but that they may find helpful. Alternatively, these behaviours may be the only ones that they have available to them at that time. There is always a reason for the behaviour. Is the behaviour a way to communicate their needs? Is the person in pain? Is the environment causing concern? Is it a strategy that has worked in the past to meet their needs or something they want? It is the job of a health professional to assess the situation and see how the situation can be best managed in the short term and constructively support the person's needs in the long term. It is beneficial for all professionals who encounter people who may exhibit challenging behaviour to have training and education in mental health so as to recognise people who may be experiencing mental health issues and to understand some of the underlying reasons for the behaviour so as to positively engage with the person in a consistent and person-centred manner.

WHAT TO DO IF THE PERSON IS SUICIDAL

When you talk to the person, try to be calm, open and honest. Try not to be judgmental, shocked or take their behaviour personally. Try to see the situation from their point of view and understand why they feel the way they do. Let the person know you support them and listen to them express their feelings. If the situation is urgent, seek help; for example, contact emergency services. If the situation is not of immediate urgency, help the person make a plan about what to do when they feel suicidal. This will help the person feel supported, safe and more in control of their situation.

Encourage the person to get support from health professionals, such as their general practitioner or a mental health professional, and offer to go with them to their appointments if they are scared or uncomfortable. Chapter 6 on assessing risk provides further detail about assessment processes with a person who is actively suicidal.

Box 7.1 (overleaf) lists the dos and don'ts with a person who is suicidal.

WHAT TO DO IF A PERSON IS SELF-HARMING

Self-harm is used to describe a range of intentional behaviours that may be hidden, impulsive or planned. This can also be known as non-suicidal self-injury. Behaviours can include:

- cutting
- burning
- scalding
- breaking bones
- swallowing drugs or objects

Box 7.1	Dos and don'ts when a person is suicidal

Do:

- stay with the person
- ask if the person is suicidal
- ask if the person has a plan
- ask if the person has any weapons (guns, knives) and their location
- ask if the person is on any medication and where those medications are
- ask if the person has taken any medications or other drugs and alcohol, and what amounts
- ask about the frequency and nature of their suicidal thoughts
- engage in conversation with a view to helping the person realise suicide is not the only or best option
- acknowledge their distress
- call for help or an ambulance if the person is bleeding or loses consciousness.

Don't:

- dismiss the person's reasons for wishing to die
- express frustration with the person
- make judgments about the person's behaviour (e.g. that they are selfish)
- tell the person they are just attention seeking
- dismiss self-harming behaviour as not requiring help and support (self-harming behaviour acts as a stress-reduction mechanism for people and is a hard pattern to break).

- hair pulling
- self-mutilation/ skin carving
- punching
- interference with wound healing.

Reasons for such behaviour are complex and can include needing to relieve stress and anxiety, punishing self, expressing anger, grief or guilt or trying to remain in control. Self-harming behaviour is a serious event, and while people who engage in these behaviours often speak of it being a way to cope, it nonetheless increases the risk for suicide. People who self-harm may also exhibit impulsive behaviours, such as binge drinking or using non-prescription substances. Remember that people who self-harm may still have suicidal thoughts, and assessment of this is required. See Box 7.2 for dos and don'ts if a person is self-harming.

WHAT TO DO WHEN WORKING WITH PEOPLE WITH A PERSONALITY DISORDER

The importance of establishing boundaries to sustain a therapeutic relationship with a person with mental illness was discussed in Chapter 3. People diagnosed with a personality disorder are often negatively labelled and the phrase 'they're just a PD' is commonly heard in health and social service settings. This involves a judgment that the person with this diagnosis is not really sick but is deliberately misbehaving or does not deserve treatment. As described in Chapter 4, people with personality disorders have legitimate mental health problems that are treatable and exhibit behaviours that are difficult or unhelpful in an effort to manage their distress. Health professionals need to take care not to engage in unhelpful behaviours themselves in reacting to stressful interpersonal situations. Clinician stigma towards these people decreases their chances of recovery.

Box 7.2   **Dos and don'ts when a person has self-harmed**

Do:

- ring an ambulance if the person has ingested poison or overdosed, has a fluctuating consciousness or is bleeding
- be calm and honest in talking to them
- keep the person physically safe
- show care and compassion
- acknowledge and treat the pain and wound if the person has been cutting.

Don't:

- take it personally
- be judgmental
- look horrified, angry or disgusted (or other signs of shock)
- tell them they are wasting your time
- tell them they need to get over themselves.

People with a personality disorder respond to supportive and consistent care that accepts their distress but that also focuses on their existing strengths and the skills they can use to manage their distress and help in their recovery. The core aim of treating people with a personality disorder is to maintain a therapeutic working relationship and to work with them to reduce their distress and facilitate better coping.

The most common type of personality disorder that health professionals will come across is the borderline type (BPD). BPD is a legitimate illness and causes significant morbidity and mortality. Despite what people think, mental health workers without advanced training can work successfully with people with BPD. Accepting the person and validating their experiences, showing empathy and consistency and taking a non-judgmental, collaborative approach to crisis management and treatment planning can result in positive outcomes. Having a clear care plan as well as a crisis management plan and close follow-up with the person is vital to assisting their recovery. Health professionals may encounter people with a paranoid personality disorder or people who have antisocial tendencies. Paranoid personality disorder may be misinterpreted as paranoid psychosis, so careful assessment is required.

See Box 7.3 for dos and don'ts for working with people with a personality disorder.

WHAT TO DO IF THE PERSON HAS EXPERIENCED AN ACUTE TRAUMA (PHYSICAL, PSYCHOLOGICAL OR SEXUAL ASSAULT)

A traumatic event can be defined as an experience that causes physical, emotional or psychological harm or distress to a person. It is an event that is perceived and experienced as a threat to one's safety or to the stability of one's world.

A traumatic event is one in which the person may have, for example:

- been involved in a traffic or physical accident
- witnessed a traffic accident
- been physically or sexually assaulted
- been mugged or robbed or have been a victim of domestic violence
- witnessed a terrible event (e.g. fire, shooting, bank hold-up, hit and run)
- been involved in severe weather events (e.g. bushfire, flood, cyclone).

People respond to such unexpected events in different ways, but in the initial phase they experience physical shock and may appear dazed and

Box 7.3	Do's and don'ts with people with a personality disorder

Do:

- have an agreed written care plan with the person for times of crisis
- have a clear management plan that the whole team agrees to, and regularly review and revise the person's goals
- be positive and maintain an attitude of hope
- set appropriate limits and boundaries about acceptable and unacceptable behaviours
- be honest and open with the person
- respond to the person, not the diagnosis/label
- set realistic and achievable goals with the person
- use clinical supervision to work on interpersonal issues associated with working with a person (Cleary & Raeburn 2017).

Don't:

- try to 'rescue' the person
- believe you are the only one who can help the person
- offer to see the person outside your working hours
- be defensive or verbally retaliate as a result of feeling 'attacked' by the person
- try to be the person's friend
- agree to keep information provided by the person secret from the rest of the multidisciplinary team
- avoid the person
- be over-controlling of the person's behaviour
- use sarcasm or cynical comments in relating with the person
- be jealous of the attention the person receives
- feel that your skills are of no worth in the care of this person.

feel numb. They may physically tremble, be very distressed or agitated, cry or wail, wander around in a confused state, or sit without appearing to realise what is happening around them. This is entirely normal in relation to what has happened to them. Box 7.4 lists the dos and don'ts if the person has experienced an acute trauma.

| **Box 7.4** | **Dos and don'ts if the person has experienced an acute trauma** |

Do:

- establish if the person has been physically hurt and needs medical attention
- talk to the person, but don't pressure them to talk
- stay with the person and reassure them that help is being arranged or is on its way
- keep the person warm
- reassure the person that what they are feeling is normal given what has happened to them.

Don't:

- minimise what has happened or what the person has witnessed
- offer the person alcohol
- tell the person to pull themselves together or that they will 'get over it'
- ask them questions repeatedly.

After the crisis has passed

After the initial shock of the trauma, people commonly experience symptoms of anxiety, fear, dizziness, breathlessness, pounding heart and insomnia. It is useful to encourage them to attend to normal daily activities as much as they can, to be as physically active as possible and to eat and drink well to promote a beneficial daily routine. Further support may be required, but most people recover on their own within a few weeks. If in doubt, the person should be encouraged to see a health professional for support.

WHAT TO DO IF THE PERSON IS AGGRESSIVE OR VIOLENT

How to tell if someone is potentially violent

If a person is angry and potentially violent, they are likely to exhibit some of the following:

- being verbally threatening or sarcastic
- being withdrawn

- dilated pupils
- furrowed brows
- grinding their teeth
- having poor concentration
- pacing or other signs of restlessness
- shouting or talking very quietly
- staring or exhibiting prolonged eye contact
- swearing
- voicing delusions or hallucinations with violent content.

Note that more than one attribute often applies.

De-escalation: act don't react!

De-escalation is a process intended to reduce tension in a situation and prevent the situation from deteriorating, therefore avoiding violence and people being hurt and traumatised. The aim is to reduce the level of tension in order for discussion to occur. De-escalation can be used in all settings. *Never* approach an angry person without back-up and do *not* attempt to restrain someone on your own, unless life is in immediate danger. Call for assistance if you need to. If you are in imminent danger, remove yourself from the situation to somewhere safe and raise the alarm.

In interactions, remember to speak slowly and calmly, in a quiet voice but loud enough to be heard. Introduce yourself to the person by saying your name and explain your actions. One person should assume control of a potentially disturbed situation. The lead person needs to manage the environment (e.g. remove bystanders, create space, direct security guards, call the police).

De-escalation is a process that involves a delimiting (creating safety) of the situation, clarification of the problem for the person and moving to a resolution (Bowers 2014). Delimiting involves conducting a safety assessment of the situation, and considering physical (not social) distancing to allow a feeling of space and safety between you and the person. Creating a quiet place away from lots of stimulus is particularly important in busy acute areas such as emergency departments. Involving supports such as security guards or police may also be used but with caution. While this may prevent a situation escalating, and can be used when additional support is required, the use of a security presence can also incite a person further. The use of assistants in nursing or healthcare workers may be more beneficial as they can be perceived as less threatening or intimidating and more likely to establish rapport and build a therapeutic relationship (Gerace et al 2018). The clarification phase involves finding out what the problem is. 'What is the matter?'-type enquiries attempt to sort out any confusion, remind the person where they are and remind them of any relationship you have with them. Find out from the person what they want. Maintain respect and empathy at all times. The resolution phase is the final stage where you can suggest a flexible approach to deal with the person's complaint and offer as many options as possible in the context of safety. Where you can't be flexible, explain why. Take your time and actively listen to the person. In some situations, reasoning is not possible, and violence will eventuate. If faced with this, safety concerns must always take precedence.

An essential component in de-escalation is to remain calm and be engaged. Body language is an important part of all communication. Try not to show your anxiety, but do show that you care. Remain self-assured without being perceived as threatening. Treating a person with respect and demonstrating compassionate care by empathising with their feelings rather than reacting to the behaviour shows genuine interest in a person and a willingness to understand why they are feeling agitated.

Box 7.5 (overleaf) lists the dos and don'ts in an aggressive or violent situation.

DEBRIEFING

After any incident, debriefing is a useful way to allow the emotions of the event to be discussed and dealt with. It is also an important process to gain insights into the sequence of events, mistakes that were made and associated learning. The purpose of debriefing is to:

- establish what happened and how people perceived the event and their level of comfort/discomfort
- make changes to prevent or reduce similar events in the future
- increase the preparedness of those being debriefed for further such incidents.

Critically reflecting on an incident allows for processing of the event. The outcome of this is personal, team and organisational development in the hope to prevent a situation arising in similar circumstances again. Being mindful of each person's role to play in a situation and what led to it occurring creates an ethical and professional workplace based on valuing each other's perspectives including the person with the lived experience of mental illness. Workplaces ought to have comprehensive debriefing processes to support staff and people in their care when unwanted events occur. It is important to check what these are where you work.

Box 7.5   Dos and don'ts in an aggressive or violent situation

Under stress, people often behave in ways that are thought to be helpful to all concerned at the time but in fact have the opposite effect and make the situation worse. The following dos and don'ts are intended to guide your interaction in situations of violence.

Body posture and eye contact

Do:

- allow the person more personal space than you might normally
- lower your voice; often the upset person will lower their voice in response
- try to relax your posture and stand at a slight angle with your arms by your sides, but make sure your stance is such that you can retreat if necessary
- make intermittent eye contact
- appear calm and genuinely interested in the person.

Don't:

- cross your arms
- stand with your legs well apart and front-on to the person
- keep your hands in your pockets
- stare at the person
- try to touch the person.

Engagement and communication

Do:

- introduce yourself by name
- speak clearly and slowly
- explain your actions
- attempt to establish rapport
- encourage the person to talk and to tell you how they view the problem
- give clear, brief instructions
- take your time (don't try to rush things along)
- emphasise your concern and desire to work together
- offer options that are realistic
- focus on the person, nod when they talk, accept their concerns as valid and demonstrate empathy

- use open questions and say 'Go on … tell me more about that …'
- match the person's arousal but not their anger (e.g. 'It sounds like we need to sort this out straightaway').

Don't:

- ask 'why' questions (they are more likely to provoke the person)
- tell the person you know how they feel (you don't)
- disagree with the person
- tell the person to calm down
- shout or talk to the person loudly (unless it is to be heard)
- make promises you cannot keep
- make threats (e.g. 'If you don't comply, you will be taken to hospital against your will/detained/secluded')
- use sarcasm, humour or minimise what they are saying (e.g. put-downs such as 'Don't be silly' or 'That's ridiculous'), which can make things worse.

WHAT TO DO IF THE PERSON IS ACUTELY PSYCHOTIC

If a person is acutely psychotic, be very clear about what the purpose of your interaction is (e.g. to establish rapport, to help them remain calm, to encourage the taking of medication, to request that they come with you to hospital, to conduct a mental state assessment, or to gain information about family so they can be informed of the person's whereabouts). It is likely that the person may be too thought-disordered to maintain concentration or stay on track in a conversation so keep sentences short and clear. It is likely they will be experiencing beliefs you do not share, therefore validate their feelings rather than argue or challenge them on the content. Box 7.6 (overleaf) lists the dos and don'ts if a person is psychotic.

WHAT TO DO IF THE PERSON IS HAVING A PANIC ATTACK

A panic attack is an episode of intense fear. It is generally triggered by negative thoughts and accompanied by one or more symptoms such as:

- chest pain
- choking

Box 7.6   **Dos and don'ts if a person is acutely psychotic**

Do:

- establish if the person is oriented
- listen to the person
- acknowledge that the person may be feeling frightened/scared/upset/angry/confused
- speak slowly, calmly and clearly
- acknowledge that what is happening is real to the person (i.e. don't try to talk them out of it or deny it is real, which is likely to make things worse)
- try to find some common ground through chatting
- say 'I know the voices are real to you'
- try to establish how much insight the person has (i.e. awareness of their illness)
- say you are trying to understand what is happening for them
- acknowledge how they are feeling (e.g. 'Those thoughts must be frightening to you').

Don't:

- argue with the person or disagree with their reality
- tell them that they are sick/mad/loony
- make glib remarks (e.g. 'You'll be right')
- tell them to pull themselves together
- express frustration.

- dizziness
- fear of dying
- fear of losing control
- heart palpitations
- intense feelings of dread
- nausea
- shortness of breath
- sweating
- trembling or shaking
- urge to escape.

Panic attacks are frightening, but fortunately they are physically harmless episodes. They can occur at random or after a person is exposed to various events that may bring on an attack. They peak in intensity very rapidly and go away with or without medical help. People experiencing panic attacks may fear they are dying, that they are suffocating or that they are having a heart attack. They may voice fears that they are 'going crazy' and seek to remove themselves from whatever situation they are in.

Some people may begin breathing very rapidly and complain that their heart is 'jumping around in their chest'. Then, within about an hour, the symptoms fade away.

People who have repeated attacks require further evaluation from a mental health professional. Panic attacks can indicate the presence of depression, panic disorder or other forms of anxiety-based illnesses (see Chapter 4).

If you are not sure whether the person is having a panic attack or a heart attack, call an ambulance and apply first aid—airway, breathing, circulation—until help arrives.

Box 7.7 lists the dos and don'ts if the person is having a panic attack.

Box 7.7 **Dos and don'ts if a person is having a panic attack**

Do:

- take some deep breaths yourself and remain calm and in an open posture
- encourage the person to take slow, deep breaths
- remind the person that the attack will pass and cannot harm them
- acknowledge their acute distress
- try to remove the person to a quiet place with some privacy
- stay with the person until they calm down.

Don't:

- rush the person in any way
- express frustration
- tell the person they are being ridiculous
- give orders
- tell the person to snap out of it or calm down (they can't)
- encourage the person to face their fears (this is not the right time).

WHAT TO DO IF THE PERSON IS INTOXICATED WITH DRUGS OR ALCOHOL

Box 7.8 lists the dos and don'ts if a person is intoxicated.

About methamphetamine intoxication

People intoxicated with methamphetamine can be unpredictable in their behaviour experiencing highly agitated states, confusion, hostility, distress, severe mood swings and, in some cases, drug-induced psychosis. This can present a serious safety risk to themselves and others, including fellow patients. Due to extreme cognitive impairment and being unable to take direction, attempts at communicating with people intoxicated can be perceived as confrontational. In some cases, sedation to reduce the risk of harming themselves may be required along with the involvement of the police or security personnel.

Box 7.8   **Dos and don'ts if a person is intoxicated**

Do:

- talk in a slow, clear and simple manner
- summon help immediately
- observe the person closely
- maintain the person's airway and breathing
- maintain the physical safety of the person and those around them
- conduct a full physical examination, including a urine screen
- assess the level of use in the past month, including the type of drug, volume, frequency and route of administration (oral, intramuscular, intravenous)
- observe closely and document for signs of withdrawal such as tremor, sweating of hands and face, insomnia, fatigue, anxiety, irritability and physical cramps.

Don't:

- attempt to engage in lengthy discussions while the person is intoxicated
- invade their personal space.

Note: Acute withdrawal requires hospital care due to the risk of seizures and severity of withdrawal symptoms.

About alcohol intoxication and withdrawal

As alcohol is consumed by populations worldwide, it is not surprising alcohol intoxication is by far one of the most common presentations to the emergency services. Though for most, drinking alcohol is not a problem, there are a significant amount of people who are injured or suffer physically and mentally from harmful drinking. Alcohol intoxication impairs both physical and mental ability. It can cause agitation, confusion, poor judgment, memory loss, slurred speech and loss of control of bodily movement (ataxia). Ultimately, it can lead to unconsciousness and death. Management of severe alcohol detoxification, i.e. those people with high blood alcohol levels, usually requires medical intervention. For the person who has a history of long-term heavy drinking withdrawal usually occurs within 24 hours of the last drink. Symptoms can include tremor ('the shakes'), increased blood pressure, sleeplessness, anxiety and loss of appetite. Some people will experience seizures within a couple of days of abstinence and therefore require close monitoring.

CONCLUSION

Behaviours of concern can involve any situation where a person is highly distressed. It will take time and education to learn how to manage such situations effectively. Appearing calm, interested and confident is the best first impression to give to a person in distress. Remember always to seek assistance from others if you are unsure what to do.

REFERENCES

Bowers, L. (2014). A model of de-escalation. *Mental Health Practice, 17*(9), 36–37.

Cleary, M., Raeburn, T. (2017). Personality disorders. In K. Evans, D. Nizette & A. O'Brien (Eds.), *Psychiatric and health nursing* (4th ed., pp. 391–407). Chatswood: Elsevier.

Gerace, A., Muir-Cochrane, E. C., O'Kane, D., et al. (2018). Assistants in nursing working with mental health consumers in the emergency department. *International Journal of Mental Health Nursing, 27*(6), 1729–1741.

WEB RESOURCES

Ambulance Tasmania De-escalation Techniques: https://www.dhhs.tas.gov.au/ambulance/community_information/handsoff/de-escalation_techniques. A quick guide to verbal de-escalation techniques for ambulance and health transport.

Bowers' de-escalation model: http://www.safewards.net/images/pdf/Talk%20Down%20poster_print%20out.pdf. A poster of 'talk down' tips for people in crisis.

Mindframe, Suicide: http://www.mindframe-media.info/for-media/reporting-suicide/facts-and-stats. Facts and statistics about suicide in Australia.

National Education Alliance of Borderline Personality Disorder Australia (NEA. BPDAust): www.bpdaustralia.com. This website provides the latest research and information from around the globe about borderline personality disorder.

Queensland MIND Essentials—Caring for a person who is aggressive or violent: https://www.health.qld.gov.au/__data/assets/pdf_file/0031/444586/aggressive. pdf. Guidelines for nurses when dealing with a person who is aggressive.

Stratis Health, Older People Mental Health Training—Prevention and de-escalation: https://www.youtube.com/watch?v=xbfeL4YiF0A.

8 TRAUMA-INFORMED CARE

INTRODUCTION

This chapter introduces the concept of trauma-informed care and how the framework can be applied in everyday practice within the context of working with people experiencing mental health issues.

Trauma-informed care is a strengths-based approach that acknowledges and understands that a significant number of people living in the community may have experienced trauma. By recognising trauma and the impact it can have on a person's wellbeing, health professionals are able to provide effective trauma-informed practice that promotes recovery. Trauma-informed practice delivered through a therapeutic relationship can reduce distress in people, increase a person's sense of wellbeing and enable the development of more-effective coping and problem-solving skills. This chapter will be useful to health practitioners and other professionals who encounter people experiencing mental health issues in their everyday practice.

TRAUMA-INFORMED CARE

Trauma-informed care has slowly evolved since the 1970s when war veterans returning from Vietnam necessitated a better professional understanding of the effects of trauma. Alongside this, advocacy campaigns promoting the voice of trauma survivors of domestic and child abuse were growing in influence. The concept continued to expand by acknowledging that trauma is widespread and can occur in anyone regardless of age, gender, ethnicity or status. Trauma can result when someone has experienced a singular traumatic event or a series of repetitive events (see Table 8.1). It could be as a result of abuse, injury, poverty, neglect, loss, violence and war; however, it is important to note that it is not the event itself that defines the trauma but how the event has impacted on a person's experience and reaction to it. A person's response to trauma is unique and individual. The psychological, and neurological effects that occur will be

TABLE 8.1
Experiences of trauma

Type of trauma	Description
Single incident trauma	Single incident trauma is sometimes described in the literature as Type I Trauma and 'relates to an unexpected and "out of the blue" event such as a natural disaster, traumatic accident, terrorist attack or single episode of assault, abuse or witnessing of such an event'.
Complex trauma	Complex trauma is sometimes described in the literature as Type II Trauma and relates to prolonged or repeated traumatic events that often begin in childhood and extend over long periods of time. Typically, the events are interpersonal, such as neglect, physical and sexual abuse. Experiences of complex trauma are prevalent in young people presenting with a broad range of psychiatric diagnoses and significantly compound the severity and complexity of these presentations.
Secondary trauma	Secondary trauma can arise when someone hears first-hand about the traumatic experience of another, for example professionals working with traumatised populations, including mental health and social workers. It can also occur through exposure to accounts of trauma by peers or the media.
Intergenerational trauma	Intergenerational trauma is the impact of trauma experienced in parents' lives being passed down to their children. Intergenerational trauma is often discussed in the context of Aboriginal and Torres Strait Islander young peoples and among children of refugees. It can also be experienced by children of veterans and other parents continuing to be affected by their own trauma.

Source: Bendall et al 2018

different for each person and their ongoing responses may vary depending on the situation. A state of high arousal brings about overwhelming stress and disrupts the ability of the brain and body to function in an integrated manner. Common emotional reactions may include extreme anxiety, anger, fear, helplessness, confusion, destructive behaviour and sadness. By being trauma aware, health professionals can work together to provide a safe and therapeutic environment that assists recovery. Trauma-informed care is now used across many service areas including social services, primary healthcare, education, youth justice and mental health.

EXPOSURE TO TRAUMA

There is a growing body of evidence showing that exposure to trauma in childhood has implications for a child's development and their emotional regulation in adulthood (Kezelman & Stavropoulos 2018). Typical development for those children unaffected by trauma involves the ability to successfully have control of their emotions and behaviour. Social, emotional and cognitive development allows them to adapt to circumstances, and thrive in most situations. Alternatively, for young children exposed to adverse and traumatic events, the brain's development is still in progress meaning other aspects of development and functioning can be delayed or altered (Kezelman & Stavropoulos 2018, McLean 2016). Neuroscience indicates this can result in poor social attachments, emotional dysregulation, language issues and behavioural difficulties that continue into adult life. Many adulthoods with a childhood experience of trauma go on to experience mental health issues in the struggle to manage their traumatic reactions and/or unhealthy coping behaviour. Neuroimaging on brain structures and functioning of those who have experienced trauma have shown neurobiological changes that signify an automatic learned response leading to a heightened alert system, often referred to as 'fight, flight or freeze response'. This alert system, in turn, can influence a person's reactions to a situation (Bendall et al 2018). It is an innate survival response where the body reacts without any conscious deliberation even on occasions when there appears no obvious threat. Health professionals can sensitively explore the trauma a child or adult has experienced and understand their response to it within the context of the presenting stimulus, behaviour, mood and thoughts in order to respond more effectively to individual needs across the lifespan.

TRAUMA AND MENTAL HEALTH

Trauma has long-term consequences. Triggers in the environment such as noises, objects or a particular visual cue can activate a response to a past traumatic event resulting in a diminished sense of control over one's emotions, thoughts and behaviour. Similarly, those with a lived experience of trauma can misinterpret social situations, exhibit behaviour that appears erratic or unpredictable and struggle to form interpersonal relationships. Such individual reactions compromise a person's ability to think clearly, make rational decisions and respond appropriately to a given situation.

Behaviour associated with hyperarousal such as shaking or sweating is easy to observe, whereas people who 'freeze' as a result of the innate survival response may be more difficult to identify. Feelings of vagueness, being on 'the outside' or 'being numb' are common terms used to describe this survival strategy. It is known as dissociation and refers to how a person assimilates information to protect themselves. A person will disconnect or detach their sense of self from a sensory experience (memories or triggers) to prevent becoming overwhelmed by emotions. The reaction is not part of their conscious awareness and has implications for day-to-day functioning. It is well known that a large proportion of people with borderline personality disorder have experienced significant adverse events in childhood, particularly sexual abuse (de Aquino Ferreira 2018, Grenyer 2019). Working in a framework of trauma-informed care allows health professionals to reframe a person's experience. Being trauma-aware accepts the chaotic feelings that may be experienced as the person struggles with their own emotions and inability to cope associated with a history of trauma. This person-centred approach is far more respectful and empathic than some of the historical and stigmatising terms often used to describe people, without trying to understand the reasons behind a person's behaviour.

PRINCIPLES OF TRAUMA-INFORMED CARE

Trauma-informed care has been established on a set of core principles that can be implemented in any setting. The principles provide a framework that can be used to deliver care as a whole-of-service philosophy rather than offering trauma-specific interventions for individuals. The aim is to not only recognise the different types of trauma people experience but to also work in a way that prevents further traumatisation. For example, in mental health services this would include the reduction of coercive and controlling practices, specifically the elimination of seclusion and restraint. Despite the use of seclusion and restraint being considered a safety measure to reduce a person's risk to self and others, it does not account for the force, nature, loss of control and experience of the individual who is subject to the intervention. Seclusion and restraint of a person is both psychologically harmful and can lead to physical injury, even death. The act itself is traumatising and can often instigate retraumatisation for those who have been subject to previous trauma in their life. Likewise, unintentional gender ratios of staffing may not allow for gender sensitivity and responsiveness in males and females to meet their gender-specific needs and ensure their physical and emotional safety.

Delivering trauma-informed care is not the responsibility of one person alone. It requires teamwork and effort on the part of an organisation (as well as individuals) to integrate the principles into all areas of service delivery including policy, procedures and protocols. For trauma-informed care to be truly effective, all staff, including administration, receptionists and other non-clinical staff should be educated on how to recognise the signs and symptoms of trauma and how to engage safely with people who are in distress. The core principles of trauma-informed care are:

1. Safety
2. Trustworthiness and transparency
3. Peer support
4. Collaboration and mutuality
5. Empowerment, voice and choice
6. Cultural, historical, and gender issues (Office of Public Health Preparedness and Response 2020)

Each principle fits well within the model of mental health recovery. They are founded on a clear evidence base, promote person-centred care through collaboration and partnerships, foster empowerment and encourage consumer and carer engagement.

IMPLEMENTING TRAUMA-INFORMED CARE

As already established trauma-informed care is not the role of one person alone. Changing the culture of a workplace takes time and effort. It involves changes in both organisational and clinical practice, therefore is implemented at a service, organisational, team and individual level. Consideration of the environment (buildings, spaces), resources, and communication strategies are key areas that can transform a service from one that can inadvertently re-traumatise a person to one that comprehends the significance of trauma and the importance of trauma-informed care.

Training and education for all professionals working with people living with mental illness will assist the implementation of trauma-informed care. Screening for trauma is also a fundamental aspect of care delivery; however, there is disagreement whether this is undertaken as part of a preliminary assessment or later once a therapeutic relationship has been established. While there is support in providing an opportunity for a person to disclose their experience of trauma to facilitate understanding, identify strengths and resources and target appropriate support needs and interventions, others argue some individuals are at risk of re-traumatisation by speaking of their experience. Ultimately, the goal is to allow time where the person feels safe to talk about the trauma in their own time. Quality practice in trauma-informed care means reframing a health professional's thinking and actions from 'what's wrong with this person?' to 'what's happened to this person?' Such a simple change of question looks beyond the behaviour being presented and attempts to understand the underlying cause and acknowledge the feelings associated with it.

ESSENTIAL SKILLS IN THE THERAPEUTIC RELATIONSHIP

Basic skills of communication are fundamental in the practice of trauma-informed care. The core principles should inform and be applicable to every interaction made by health professionals. See Box 8.1. Communication is the key to any successful therapeutic relationship. Listening and knowing how to listen attentively (active listening) sends the message to the person that you are hearing them and acknowledging/accepting what they are saying. This technique builds empathy and increases understanding. When a health professional demonstrates a calm, reliable, respectful and consistent approach, it can assist a person to regulate their own emotions and feel in control of what's happening in the environment around them. Helping the person identify the issue or problem and focusing on their strengths and resources will support a positive outcome and prevent the occurrence of further traumatisation.

Communication skills are vital in establishing, maintaining and responding to people. They are vital in the provision of counselling. Counselling plays a significant part in the recovery of a person who has experienced trauma. There are several specific counselling therapies that can be undertaken with individuals or in groups and generally involve:

- talking, which is the vehicle to help a person to understand themselves better and/or to change unwanted or unhelpful thoughts or behaviours
- specific time set aside to talk in a comfortable, quiet place
- other techniques to help people to overcome trauma, stress, emotional problems, relationship problems or troublesome habits (e.g. excessive worrying or excessive anxiety) and gain insight (see Appendix 3).

CONCLUSION

The impact and effectiveness of trauma-informed care cannot be underestimated; a novice practitioner can be a great support just by listening and validating the person and their story. Implementing trauma-informed

---

| **Box 8.1** | Tips for trauma-informed communication |

- 'Choose your moment' if you are initiating the contact.
- Honour the person's preferences regarding the time, location for the conversation, etc., if you can.
- Your approach and style should be empathic at all times.
- Attune into their verbal and non-verbal communication.
- Consider what may have happened to the person rather than what is 'wrong' with them.
- Recognise that a person's 'challenging' behaviours and responses may be their attempts to protect themselves and to cope with stress.
- Listen to and validate the person (don't 'talk over' them or contradict them).
- Recognise the signs of stress (which may take the form of visible agitation, such as accelerated pace, raised voice or silence, glazed expression and 'shut down').
- If the person initially says they are 'okay', but you are still concerned, you can gently ask a second time as the first response may be automatic. Do not persist if the person is reluctant or insistent.
- Don't give advice unless you are asked for it (e.g. avoid saying 'Have you tried...?')
- Enquire about who the person might contact for support. Provide contact numbers for any relevant services or where to find them if necessary.
- Ensure the person does not leave the conversation in a distressed state.

Source: Kezelman & Stavropoulos 2018, pp. 90–91

---

care and awareness into organisational culture, practices and policies will allow health professionals to recognise, respond and support a person in their recovery. Experience and education in the area will enable the practitioner to have increased therapeutic capacity to engage with a person who has experienced trauma with compassion, empathy, understanding and respect.

REFERENCES

Bendall, S., Phelps, A., Browne, V., et al. (2018) *Trauma and young people: moving toward trauma-informed services and systems*. Melbourne: Orygen, The National Centre of Excellence in Youth Mental Health.

de Aquino Ferreira, L.F., Queiroz Pereira, F.H., Neri Benevides, A.M.L., Aguiar Melo, M.C. (2018) Borderline personality disorder and sexual abuse: a systematic review. *Psychiatry Research,* Apr; *262,* 70-77.

Grenyer, B. (2019). Integrating trauma-informed care for personality disorders – The Project Air Strategy. In R. Benjamin, J. Haliburn & S. King (Eds.). *Humanising mental health care in Australia*, pp. 380–391. London: Routledge.

Kezelman C.A & Stavropoulos P.A. (2018) *Talking about trauma: guide to conversations and screening for health and other service providers.* Sydney: Blue Knot Foundation.

McLean S. (2016) *The effect of trauma on the brain development of children—evidence-based principles for supporting the recovery of children in care*. Melbourne: Australian Institute of Family Studies.

Office of Public Health Preparedness and Response (2020) *6 guiding principles to a trauma-informed approach.* Centre for Preparedness and Response. Online. Available: https://www.cdc.gov/cpr/infographics/6_principles_trauma_info.htm 8 March 2021.

WEB RESOURCES

Blue Knot Foundation—Supporting adult survivors of childhood trauma & abuse: https://www.blueknot.org.au/. The Blue Knot Foundation is a leading source for training, resources and information for consumers, carers and services.

Hagar New Zealand—the whole journey: https://hagar.org.nz/trauma-informed-care/ this website offers support for women and children experiencing trauma as a result of slavery, human trafficking and abuse.

Substance Abuse and Mental Health Services Administration (SAMHSA) (2014). *Concept of trauma and guidance for a trauma-informed approach.* HHS Publication No. (SMA) 14-4884. Rockville, MD: SAMHSA. Online. Available: https://ncsacw.samhsa.gov/userfiles/files/SAMHSA_Trauma.pdf 8 March 2021. This paper offers a framework to develop a working concept of trauma and a trauma-informed approach.

TheRoyalAustralianandNewZealandCollegeofPsychiatrists–Trauma-informedpractice:| https://www.ranzcp.org/news-policy/policy-and-advocacy/position-statements/ trauma-informed-practice. This is a position statement to assert the importance of trauma-informed care and to reduce re-traumatisation.

INTRODUCTION

Psychiatric medications, sometimes referred to as psychotropic medications, are prescribed by health professionals including psychiatrists, general practitioners and nurse practitioners authorised to dispense medications to treat symptoms of mental illness. This chapter describes commonly used medications to treat symptoms and associated side effects, general management issues for health professionals, such as concordance (compliance/adherence) with medication regimens, and outlines the difficulties facing people required to take these medicines for long periods of time. The information contained in this chapter will also be useful in advising carers about the responsibilities they may have regarding medications for a person they are supporting.

Recently, the effectiveness of psychiatric medications—in particular, antidepressants—has been challenged. However, many of these medications remain a useful treatment option for people. While non-pharmacological interventions should always be considered a first-line treatment option, psychiatric medications can be used as a short- or long-term intervention, and in combination with other psychological-based treatments. The decision to use medication is often based on a comprehensive assessment, the severity and type of illness being experienced, and consideration of what is best to promote recovery, including a person's consent in the decision-making process.

CATEGORIES OF MEDICATION

There are four essential pharmacological categories of medication used to treat mental illness:

- anxiolytics (anti-anxiety drugs)
- antidepressants
- antipsychotics
- mood stabilisers.

Medications can have two names—the generic name (i.e. the active compound of the drug) and the trade name (i.e. the registered brand name given by a particular drug company). For example, diazepam is the name of the actual drug, but Valium is a brand name for this drug. In some countries, generic-named medications can be cheaper than their brand-name counterparts. In this chapter, the generic name is listed first, with the brand name in parentheses.

Anxiolytics

Anxiolytics are used primarily in emergency and mental health settings for relieving acute panic and anxiety, insomnia, obsessive-compulsive disorder and alcohol withdrawal. Diazepam is the most well-known anxiolytic. It belongs to the benzodiazepine family. These drugs are often colloquially referred to as 'benzos'. They act by enhancing the effects of GABA (gamma-aminobutyric acid), a neurotransmitter in the central nervous system.

Other commonly used anxiolytics can be found in Table 9.1.

In small doses, these drugs have a calming and slowing-down effect; in high doses, they are sedating. Side effects are common and include headache, nausea, hypotension (low blood pressure) and unsteadiness. People taking anxiolytics are encouraged to take care when driving or operating machinery. Anxiolytics may also be used to treat acute psychosis in psychiatric wards as an adjunct to antipsychotics. Anxiolytics are sometimes used in the acute phase of delirium as well.

TABLE 9.1
Commonly used anxiolytic medication

Generic name	Brand name
Alprazolam	Xanax, Kalma, Alprax
Temazepam	Normison, Temtabs, Temaze
Nitrazepam	Mogadon, Alodorm
Oxazepam	Serepax, Oxanid, Serax
Bromazepam	Lexotan, Lectopam
Clonazepam	Rivotril, Paxam
Flunitrazepam	Rohypnol, Hypnodorm
Lorazepam	Ativan, Almazine
Triazolam	Halcion, Trilam

In the short term these drugs relieve anxiety and insomnia but should only be prescribed for two to three weeks because of the risk of dependency. Further, higher doses are required over time to achieve an equivalent initial therapeutic effect. Abrupt discontinuation can result in increased anxiety, sleep disturbance, irritability, increased anxiety, hand tremor, sweating, concentration problems, aching limbs and nausea, which can be very unpleasant. Withdrawal from long-term use requires medical supervision and should be gradual to avoid difficult withdrawal symptoms. The serious side effects listed in Box 9.1 are often seen in people taking benzodiazepines for long periods of time. Often people have started these drugs without having been prescribed them by a health professional.

Drug interactions
Benzodiazepines can be dangerous when combined with other drugs such as alcohol or methadone. These can potentiate the respiratory depressant effect of benzodiazepines, which sometimes results in vomiting, respiratory obstruction and death.

Antidepressants

Antidepressants are used to relieve depressive symptoms including suicidal thoughts and feelings. They are also prescribed to treat anxiety, panic disorder and obsessive-compulsive disorder. There is an array of antidepressants available today in four main groups:

- selective serotonin reuptake inhibitors (SSRIs)
- serotonin and noradrenaline reuptake inhibitors (SNRIs)

Box 9.1   Side effects of Anxiolytics

Side effects include:

- drug dependency (i.e. being unable to stop taking the drug)
- impaired memory and concentration
- sedation
- feelings of being 'cut off' from one's own feelings
- low mood
- poor motor coordination
- mood swings, irritability and anger.

- tricyclics—an older group and less commonly prescribed today
- monoamine oxidase inhibitors (MAOIs)—an older group, uncommonly prescribed today.
  Antidepressants are prescribed for the following conditions:
- moderate to severe depression
- severe anxiety and panic attacks
- the depressed phase of a bipolar episode
- obsessive-compulsive disorders
- chronic pain
- eating disorders
- post-traumatic stress disorder.

Antidepressants are not necessary for people experiencing a mild depression or a normal grief reaction after the death of a loved one. Such experiences are understood to be within the normal range of behaviour given a major loss. However, if depression persists beyond a four- to six-month period, assessment and treatment is advised. Commonly used antidepressant medications are listed in Table 9.2.

Selective Serotonin Reuptake Inhibitors

SSRIs are believed to work by preventing the reuptake of serotonin (5-hydroxytryptamine or '5-HT') in the central nervous system. Side effects of SSRIs include nausea, diarrhoea, agitation and headaches. Serotonin syndrome is a potentially life-threatening emergency resulting from excessive serotonin activity (see Box 9.2).

Serotonin and Noradrenaline Reuptake Inhibitors

SNRIs are a relatively new form of antidepressant that work on both noradrenaline and 5-HT neurotransmitters. They typically have similar

TABLE 9.2
Commonly used antidepressant medications

Generic name	Brand name	Group
Fluoxetine	Prozac	SSRI
Paroxetine	Aropax	SSRI
Venlafaxine	Efexor	SNRI
Reboxetine	Edronax	SNRI
Amitriptyline	Endep	Tricyclic

> **Box 9.2** Serotonin syndrome
>
> Serotonin syndrome, a potentially life-threatening emergency resulting from excessive serotonin activity, can result from other antidepressants being combined with SSRIs (e.g. MAOIs) or being administered while the person is taking St John's wort. Overdose of a single antidepressant can also cause this syndrome. Serotonin syndrome can lead to hyperthermia (overheating), kidney failure and death if left untreated. Emergency interventions include ceasing administration of SSRIs and administering anticonvulsants and clonazepam to reduce agitation and induce calm. Taking amphetamines such as MDMA ('ecstasy') while also taking SSRIs can result in serotonin syndrome. Symptoms of serotonin syndrome are:
>
> - confusion
> - mania
> - agitation, restlessness
> - sweating
> - an urgent need to urinate and frequently
> - tremor
> - nausea
> - diarrhoea
> - headache.

side effects to SSRIs and may require a slow reduction in dosage before the drug is ceased to prevent a withdrawal syndrome.

Sexual side effects, such as loss of libido, failure to reach orgasm and erectile dysfunction, are also common.

Antidepressant Discontinuation Syndrome.

If people stop taking antidepressants abruptly a range of distressing but non-life-threatening symptoms may be experienced. The following medications appear to be associated with this syndrome: citalopram (Celexa), escitalopram (Lexapro), fluoxetine (Prozac), fluvoxamine (Luvox), paroxetine (Aropax) and sertraline (Zoloft).

Symptoms may include a flu-like reaction, as well as a variety of physical symptoms—headache, gastrointestinal distress, faintness and strange sensations of vision or touch. Sometimes people also experience anxiety and lowness of mood, which makes it hard to differentiate whether a person is becoming ill again or has discontinuation symptoms. It is very important to explain to people considering reducing or coming off their medication that they need the support of their medical and nursing staff in tailoring a reduction slowly, over time. Discontinuation symptoms can also be experienced when reducing or ceasing SNRIs.

Cyclic antidepressants

Cyclic antidepressants including tricyclics and tetracyclic medications are one of the earliest antidepressants developed. While effective, they have largely been replaced with better tolerated antidepressants that have far fewer side effects, therefore their use has greatly decreased. The mode of action for cyclic medication is thought to be due to their blockade of the reuptake of the neurotransmitters noradrenaline and serotonin in the central nervous system. More-recent drugs are more selective in blocking specific neurotransmitters, have fewer side effects and are less risky if a person were to overdose, and so are more likely to be used as a first choice of antidepressant. However, tricyclics remain the drug of choice for some people, especially those who have responded well to them, have a serious depressive illness, and who experience few bothersome side effects. Side effects include increased heart rate, drowsiness, dry mouth, constipation, urinary retention, blurred vision, dizziness, seizures and confusion. Tricyclics are toxic so can be lethal in overdose. Tricyclic toxicity is a *medical emergency* with cardiotoxic effects leading to dysrhythmias requiring immediate medical intervention. Box 9.3 lists the major signs of tricyclic overdose.

Monoamine Oxidase Inhibitors

MAOIs are rarely prescribed today because they induce a life-threatening high blood pressure interaction with foods containing tyramine (e.g. aged

---

Box 9.3   Signs of tricyclic overdose

Signs include:

- agitation
- confusion
- drowsiness
- bowel and bladder paralysis
- dysregulation of body temperature and blood pressure
- dilated pupils.

Source: Elder et al 2011

---

cheeses, red wine, broad beans), so require a special diet. MAOIs may be used as a last resort if no other medications have been useful. Their mode of action is by blocking the enzyme monoamine oxidase, which breaks down the neurotransmitters dopamine, serotonin and noradrenaline. Health professionals are more likely to encounter older people who are taking tricyclics and MAOIs because they have been effective for them in the past or they have been taking them for a long time. Side effects include dry mouth, sedation, constipation, hypotension, seizures and urinary retention.

Antipsychotics

Antipsychotics can be prescribed for treating symptoms of psychosis. Recommended for managing acute epsiodes and sustained remission of psychotic symptoms, antipsychotics are often used with people diagnosed with schizophrenia or bipolar disorder. Over the past 20 years new antipsychotics, often known as atypicals or second-generation antipsychotics, have been introduced; these have equal efficacy to the traditional antipsychotics (typical or first-generation antipsychotics), yet they have fewer but different side effects. See Table 9.3 for a list of common antipsychotic medication.

How antipsychotics work

Antipsychotics reduce or eliminate delusions, hallucinations, abnormal mood and thought disorders. They also reduce the likelihood of further

TABLE 9.3
First-generation and second-generation antipsychotics

	Generic name	Brand name
Typical or first-generation antipsychotics (less frequently used now)	Chlorpromazine	Largactil
	Haloperidol	Serenace
	Trifluoperazine	Stelazine
Atypical or second-generation antipsychotics (first-choice drugs)	Aripiprazole	Abilify
	Amisulpride	Solian
	Clozapine	Clozaril
	Olanzapine	Zyprexa
	Quetiapine	Seroquel
	Risperidone	Risperdal

episodes of psychosis. Their mode of action is blockage of dopamine and 5-HT$_{2A}$ receptors within the central nervous system. However, because these drugs work on other dopaminergic pathways in the brain, a range of unpleasant motor (movement) side effects can be experienced, known as extrapyramidal side effects (EPSEs), particularly experienced when using typical antipsychotics (see Table 9.4). In the short term, anticholinergics may be used to prevent or treat EPSE, however the efficacy base of these remains uncertain and therefore should not be used as a long-term management strategy (WHO 2012). Acute extrapyramidal side effects can be reversed or reduced with dose reduction or discontinuation. Health professionals are well placed to assess for abnormal movement disorders and to implement appropriate management strategies.

Side effects

Commonly reported intolerable side effects of antipsychotic medication as reported by users include sedation, feeling tired, unmotivated, emotional bluntness, sexual dysfunction and substantial weight gain (Bjornestad et al 2020). Other side effects can include sensitivity to sunburn, dry mouth, constipation, nausea and postural hypotension. While all antipsychotic medication can be attributed to weight gain, atypical antipsychotics (clozapine, olanzapine, risperidone) show acute weight gain, caused by craving and never feeling full after eating. This places a person at risk of metabolic syndrome, diabetes and cardiovascular disease. When the side effects are measured against the potential benefits of the medication, it is easy to appreciate why some people are hesitant to follow a prescribed treatment regime. To ensure a person is maintaining a good quality of life and as part of their recovery journey, a change of medication may be called for to alleviate the side effects. Drug holidays and psychological interventions can also be used to ameliorate side effects.

For those few diagnosed with schizophrenia who do not respond to commonly prescribed antipsychotic medication with little alleviation of the symptoms, Clozapine may be considered. Clozapine is an atypical antipsychotic but has a high risk of serious side effects.

One of the most critical side effects of clozapine is agranulocytosis (affects 1–2% of people). Regular blood screening is required—weekly for 18 weeks and monthly thereafter. Other serious risks include seizures, heart inflammation and high blood sugar levels. It should not be used in people with dementia. Clozapine interacts with many other drugs so careful monitoring of clozapine is required as serious side effects can occur with particular attention to the signs of clozapine toxicity that can lead to seizures, hypoventilation, heart arrythmias and ultimately loss of life. See Box 9.4.

TABLE 9.4
Extrapyramidal side effects of antipsychotics

Extrapyramidal side effect	Signs and symptoms	Prevalence (with older drugs)	Time it takes to develop	Treatment
Dystonia	Muscular spasm in any part of the body such as eyes rolling upwards (oculogyric crisis). Head and neck twisted (torticollis). In extreme cases, the back may arch or the jaw may dislocate. Acute dystonia can be both painful and frightening. Person may need assistance breathing.	Approximately 10%, but more common in young males, in the neuroleptic-naïve and with high-potency drugs (e.g. haloperidol). Dystonic reactions are rare in the elderly.	Acute dystonia can occur within hours of starting antipsychotics (minutes for intramuscular or intravenous use). Tardive dystonia occurs after months to years of antipsychotic treatment.	Anticholinergic drugs given orally, intramuscularly or intravenously, depending on the severity of symptoms (remember the person may be unable to swallow). Response to intravenous administration will be seen in five minutes. Response to intramuscular administration takes around 20 minutes.
Parkinsonism	Tremor and/or rigidity. Bradykinesia (decreased facial expression, flat monotone voice, slow body movements, inability to initiate movement). Bradyphrenia (slowed thinking). Salivation Parkinsonism can be mistaken for depression or the negative symptoms of schizophrenia.	Approximately 20%, but more common in elderly females and those with pre-existing neurological damage (e.g. head injury, stroke).	Days to weeks after antipsychotic drugs are started or the dose is increased.	Several options are available depending on the clinical circumstances: reduce the antipsychotic dose; change to an atypical drug; or prescribe an anticholinergic medication.

Continued

TABLE 9.4
Extrapyramidal side effects of antipsychotics—cont'd

Extrapyramidal side effect	Signs and symptoms	Prevalence (with older drugs)	Time it takes to develop	Treatment
Akathisia	A subjectively unpleasant state of inner restlessness where there is a strong desire or compulsion to move. Foot tapping when seated. Constantly crossing/uncrossing legs. Rocking from foot to foot. Constantly pacing up and down. Akathisia can be mistaken for psychotic agitation and has been linked with suicide and aggression towards others. Sometimes mistaken for anxiety.	Approximately 25%.	Acute akathisia occurs within hours to weeks of starting antipsychotics or increasing the dose. Tardive akathisia takes longer to develop and can persist after antipsychotics are withdrawn.	Reduce antipsychotic dose. Change to an atypical antipsychotic. Low-dose benzodiazepine.
Tardive dyskinesia	A wide range of movements can occur such as lip smacking or chewing, tongue protrusion, choreiform movements (pill rolling or piano playing) and pelvic thrusting. Severe orofacial movements can lead to difficulty speaking, eating or breathing. Movements are worse under stress.	5% of people per year of antipsychotic exposure. More common in elderly women, those with affective illness and those who have had acute EPSEs early on in treatment.	Months to years. Approximately 50% of cases are reversible.	Stop anticholinergic if prescribed. Reduce dose of antipsychotic. Change to atypical drug. Clozapine is the most likely drug to be associated with resolution of symptoms. Other drugs such as valproate and clonazepam may be prescribed, but evidence is poor.

Box 9.4	Recognising clozapine toxicity

Symptoms include the following.

- Confusion
- Excessive sedation
- Deliriuim
- Hypersalivation
- Blurred vision
- Fever
- Sweating
- Myoclonus (spasmodic muscle contractions)
- Rapid heartbeat
- Muscle weakness

Source: Adapted from SA Health 2017

Neuroleptic Malignant Syndrome

This is a condition where the person develops stiffness and fever, usually after beginning antispychotics. It requires immediate medical attention, hospital observation and maintenance of adequate hydration.

TOOLS FOR ASSESSING SIDE EFFECTS OF MEDICATIONS

Assessment tools include:

- the LUNSERS (Liverpool University Neuroleptic Side Effect Rating Scale) (Day et al 1995)
- the AIMS (Abnormal Involuntary Movements Scale), which is a widely used tool for use with people on long-term antipsychotic medications and is designed to assess for signs of tardive dyskinesia (see <http://www.cqaimh.org/pdf/tool_aims.pdf>)
- GASS (The Glasgow Antipsychotic Side-effect Scale) (Waddell & Taylor 2008)
- SMARTS (Systematic Monitoring of Adverse events Related to TreatmentS): The development of a pragmatic patient-completed checklist to assess antipsychotic drug side effects (Haddad et al. 2014).

Depot antipsychotic medication

Depot medication is a long-term (two to four weeks) medication that is given to those who are reluctant or unable to maintain a daily regimen of taking medication orally. Depot medication is administered by deep intramuscular injection into the ventrogluteal area using a Z-track technique according to the manufacturer's recommendations (Shepherd 2018). The injection site needs to be rotated to avoid long-term damage to the area (Yilmaz et al 2016). Those coming off depot medication need to be monitored closely because the effects of discontinuation will be delayed. Common depot medications include:

- flupenthixol decanoate (Depixol)
- fluphenazine decanoate (Modecate)
- zuclopenthixol decanoate (Clopixol)
- risperidone (Risperdal).

Shared decision making

Before commencing any treatment, information should always be provided on the possible side effects of medication and be assured it is understood by all parties involved. People receiving antipsychotic medication should be involved in treatment decisions with their own preference being heard and respected. Similarly, when a person starts taking antipsychotics, health professionals have a responsibility to provide education, monitoring and ongoing support. For instance, working in partnership with a physiotherapist, exercise physiologist and dietician can facilitate effective weight management. The important message is that there is not one type of antipsychotic medication suitable for all, and each person should be assessed individually for response and tolerability to a specific drug.

MOOD STABILISERS

Mood stabilisers are the medications prescribed to maintain a balanced mood for people with intense or shifting moods. Lithium (carbonate), a naturally occurring salt, is used in treating acute mania and for the ongoing maintenance of those with a history of mania, as is sodium valproate. Just how lithium works is not clear, but it is known to mimic the effect of sodium, thereby compromising the ability of neurons to release, activate or respond to neurotransmitters. Some of the anticonvulsants, such as sodium valproate (Epilim), carbamazepine (Tegretol) and lamotrigine (Lamictal), are also commonly used as mood stabilisers, particularly in bipolar disorder.

Box 9.5 lists common side effects of mood stabilisers.

| Box 9.5 | Side effects of mood stabilisers |

Common side effects include:

- sleepiness
- dizziness
- a metallic taste in the mouth
- increased appetite and weight gain
- a feeling of sickness, nausea
- skin rashes
- changes in blood count
- irregular menstrual periods in females.

Very rare side effects include:

- pancreatitis (less than one in 10,000 cases)
- abdominal pain, nausea and vomiting
- liver failure (less than one in 50,000 cases)
- weakness, loss of appetite, lethargy and drowsiness.

The therapeutic range for lithium is 0.6–1.2 mmol/L for acute mania and 0.6–0.8 mmol/L for maintenance, but more conservative levels are increasingly being used. Symptoms of lithium toxicity rarely appear at levels below 1.2 mmol/L but are common above 2.0 mmol/L. Therefore, as the therapeutic and toxic levels are so close, extreme care must be taken in monitoring the person's blood level regularly, especially during the early phases of treatment. If the level exceeds 1.5 mmol/L, the next dose should be withheld and a doctor notified. Levels are usually monitored weekly until stable, and then monthly.

Box 9.6 lists signs of lithium toxicity. Lithium toxicity is a *medical emergency* and requires immediate medical intervention (i.e. call an ambulance). It is important to educate about the side effects and signs of toxicity. Users must be informed of the need for regular blood-level testing. Also encourage users to drink about 10 glasses of water every day, and ensure they know to take their medication regularly, even when they are feeling well, and that machinery should not be operated until the initial drowsiness subsides. If relevant, also discuss the risks of taking lithium during pregnancy.

Box 9.6   **Signs of lithium toxicity**

Signs of lithium toxicity **in the early stages** include:

- anorexia
- nausea
- vomiting
- diarrhoea
- coarse hand tremor
- twitching
- lethargy
- slurred speech
- hyperactive deep tendon reflexes
- ataxia
- tinnitus
- vertigo
- weakness
- drowsiness.

Signs of lithium toxicity **in the later stages** include:

- fever
- decreased urinary output
- decreased blood pressure
- irregular pulse
- electrocardiograph changes
- impaired consciousness, seizures and coma.

Lithium toxicity can be a life-threatening event.

Anticonvulsants

A number of anticonvulsant drugs have also been used to treat mania, especially when lithium is ineffective. These drugs are now rapidly becoming the drug of choice for many people. Carbamazepine, valproate and topiramate are examples of commonly used anticonvulsants. These drugs have been found to have acute antimanic and mood-stabilising effects. They are not, however, antidepressants. Box 9.7 lists side effects of anticonvulsants.

Box 9.7	Side effects of anticonvulsants

Side effects include:

- *carbamazepine:* blood dyscrasias, drowsiness, nausea, vomiting, constipation or diarrhoea, hives or skin rashes and hepatitis
- *valproate:* prolonged bleeding time, gastrointestinal tract upset, tremor, ataxia, somnolence, dizziness and hepatic failure
- *topiramate:* cognitive impairment, sedation, nausea, weight loss, dizziness, vomiting, rash, agitation and paraesthesias.

DRUGS USED TO MANAGE DEMENTIA

There are different medications and treatment regimens for dementia. Medications cannot halt the progress of dementia but merely slow its progression. For a short period of time these drugs can be effective to improve quality of life for the person experiencing dementia and reduce carer burden by reducing cognitive symptoms and providing symptomatic relief.

The main types of cholinesterase inhibitor that can be used are:

- donepezil (Aricept)
- rivastigmine (Exelon)
- galantamine (Reminyl).

Other drugs include memantine (Namenda) and risperidone (Risperdal). These medications are prescribed to treat symptoms related to memory, language, judgment and thinking, but there is no cure. Cardiac conditions can be worsened by these drugs, so regular heart monitoring is required. A range of non-pharmacological interventions can support the person with dementia and their family to reduce symptoms and improve quality of life. These include behavioural, environmental and psychological strategies.

PRN MEDICATION

PRN ('as needed') medication is used as an adjunct to medication treatment in managing acutely unwell people when they are agitated or distressed due to the severity of their symptoms. PRN medication should only be given after alternative interventions such as helping the person with self-soothing strategies have been tried. Common reasons for administering PRN medication include irritability, self-harming behaviour, distressed mood, agitation, threatening behaviour, insomnia and at the person's request hence commonly administered medications

---

Box 9.8   Principles of good practice: PRN

- Remain focused on the needs of the person.
- Include PRN as part of the clinical management plan.
- Review prescriptions regularly.
- Keep rigorous documentation about the reasons for and effects of PRN.
- Train all staff in the use of PRN.
- Use PRN as a last resort.

Adapted from Baker 2016

---

in this form are antipsychotics, benzodiazepines and sleeping tablets. PRN medication can be given orally or by intramuscular injection with the user being monitored for mental and physical status after administration.

It is worth noting that while the aim of offering PRN medication may be to calm the person emotionally and to settle behaviour, it has the potential to be overused by those health professionals who administer it. It can ultimately elicit further distress in a person if they feel they have not had a choice in the matter, which, in turn, can lead to the use of coercive interventions being implemented. There is no clear theoretical basis for administering PRN medication, and care should be person-centred and with the person's involvement. Principles of good practice for using PRN are listed in Box 9.8.

GENERAL MANAGEMENT ISSUES

Taking medicines every day for more than a few days is difficult for most people to do. People with a mental illness, however, are no more likely not to take their medications than the general public. People with chronic or enduring illness such as diabetes and hypertension (high blood pressure) also have difficulty in taking medications regularly but face dire health consequences when they stop taking, or forget to take, their regular doses. Tips to assist those taking psychiatric medications are listed in Appendix 4.

Medication concordance refers to a person adhering to a specified regimen of taking medication. Medication non-concordance is one of the most common reasons for recurrence of psychotic symptoms and readmission to hospital. Health professionals are best placed to support a person in their recovery and medication regimen by discussing the reasons behind the reluctance in the first instance. There are many reasons why people discontinue psychiatric medications or refuse to take them. For example, a person may:

- feel confused, or anxious about the medication
- not think they are ill
- forget to take their medication
- believe they are better and do not need their medication anymore
- mistrust health professionals
- experience or have experienced uncomfortable, disabling or frightening side effects
- think the medication has not worked quickly enough
- not have the money to buy medication, run out of or lose their medication or have their medication stolen
- have friends and family telling them they do not need medication
- be ashamed of having an illness and don't want to be seen as weak
- be homeless and have difficulty storing or establishing a routine to remember to take their medication
- sell their medication on the street to make money.

Each of the above reasons is real and logical to the person involved, and such feelings need to be taken seriously and talked through. Making negative judgments about people taking or not taking psychiatric medications raises barriers between health professionals and those with whom they work. Box 9.9 lists questions that the person can be asked when assessing medication management, and Box 9.10 lists strategies for medication concordance.

SPECIAL POPULATIONS
Pregnancy and breastfeeding

The major period for teratogenic (drug-induced and abnormal) effects in an unborn child is the first eight weeks of gestation. Difficult ethical issues involve weighing the health of the mother in relation to the risk for the unborn child. Specialised medical advice needs to be provided to women who are pregnant or breastfeeding and experiencing symptoms of mental illness. Breastfeeding may not need to be discontinued (e.g. if there is insufficient evidence that it will harm the baby), but such a decision needs to be made by specialist medical staff.

Box 9.9   Assessment of medication management

Questions to ask the person directly include:

- What type of medication are you on?
- What is the dose?
- How often is the medication supposed to be taken?
- When do you take it?
- What does it do?
- What side effects are there?
- Do you alter the doses or do you follow the prescription exactly?
- Are you on any over-the-counter (OTC) medications? (Note that some OTC medications such as St John's wort, and cough and cold medicines cannot be taken when a person is on psychiatric medication.)

Observe the person for their ability to:

- read the directions on the medicine container
- see the pills
- discriminate between pills of a different colour
- handle the pills
- count out the pills or measure liquids
- remember the regimen.

Younger people

Prescribing medications to treat mental health problems in children and adolescents is controversial. While most medications used are safe and effective there are some central concerns including efficacy, long-term use and the effect on normal growth and development. Providing information on the medication, exploring treatment options and working in partnership with children, young people and their families allows informed choices to be made that will provide an effective pathway to recovery.

Older people

Both the physiological changes of ageing and existing medical conditions complicate the administration of medications to this population. Reduced cardiac output and reduced liver and kidney function can affect the transport and absorption of medications, in turn affecting

---

Box 9.10   Strategies to encourage medication concordance

- Spend time establishing how the person feels about medications and their illness.
- Tailor the medication regimen to the person's schedule.
- Educate the person about self-monitoring of symptoms and side effects of the medication.
- Give the person a medication container (dosette) and show them how to use it.
- Establish regular contact with the person.
- Establish what factors would motivate concordance (e.g. being able to work, engage in community activities, socialise).
- Examine what factors inhibit taking medication (e.g. uncomfortable side effects such as nausea, visible side effects such as tremor of the hands).
- Encourage the person to have regular contact with their general practitioner for health check-ups and the mental health treating team for monitoring.
- Provide information about individual-oriented and recovery-oriented groups and associations for the person to access.
- Provide education in verbal and written form to the person in small amounts and frequently.
- Encourage the person to ask questions and request more information.
- Provide information to the person's family, carers and friends about medications and side effects, and about the importance of medications in maintaining wellness.

---

efficacy. Older people tend to be more sensitive than younger adults to a number of psychiatric medications, so prescription needs to be tailored to the minimum dose with the maximum effect and fewest side effects. Risks associated with polypharmacy (where a person is on a number of medications for different conditions) can include increased risk of falls, adverse medication reactions and a reduction in the accurate diagnosis of mental illness.

CONCLUSION

This chapter has provided an overview of common medications used to treat mental illness. It is important to work with the person regarding them taking the right drug at the right time to maintain wellness. An acute awareness of the side effects and risks of taking psychiatric medications is a vital aspect of the knowledge and skills of all health workers caring for people with mental health problems.

REFERENCES

Baker, J. (2016). *Cochrane find no evidence for as required PRN medication for mental health inpatients.* Online. Available: https://www.nationalelfservice.net/treatment/medicine/cochrane-find-no-evidence-for-as-required-PRN-medication-for-mental-health-inpatients/ 26 Nov 2020.

Bjornestad, J., Lavik, K., Davidson, L., et al. (2020) Antipsychotic treatment – a systematic literature review and meta-analysis of qualitative studies. *Journal of Mental Health, 29*(5), 513–523.

Day J., Wood G., Dewey M., & Bentall R. (1995). A self-rating scale for measuring neuroleptic side-effects: validation in a group of schizophrenic patients. *British Journal of Psychiatry, 166*(5): 650–653.

Elder, R., Evans, K., & Nizette, D. (Eds.). (2011). *Psychiatric and mental health nursing* (2nd ed.). Sydney: Elsevier.

Haddad, P.M., Fleischhacker, W.W., Peuskens, J. et al. (2014) SMARTS (Systematic Monitoring of Adverse events Related to TreatmentS): The development of a pragmatic patient-completed checklist to assess antipsychotic drug side effects. *Therapeutic Advances in Psychopharmacology, 4*(1): 15–21.

SA Health. (2017). Clozapine Toxicity and Therapeutic Drug Monitoring. Online. Available: https://www.sahealth.sa.gov.au/wps/wcm/connect/dd4e7c1d-0ec2-45ad-acf4-faf849aa518b/Fact+Sheet+-+Clozapine+Toxicity+and+Therapeutic+Drug+Monitoring.pdf?MOD=AJPERES&CACHEID=ROOTWORKSPACE-dd4e7c1d-0ec2-45ad-acf4-faf849aa518b-niQkEdv 11 Nov 2020.

Shepherd, E. (2018). Injection technique 1: administering drugs via the intramuscular route. *Nursing Times* [online], *114*(8), 23–25.

Usher, K. (2017). Psychopharmacology. In K. Evans, D. Nizette, & A. O'Brien (Eds.), *Psychiatric and mental health nursing* (4th ed.). Sydney: Elsevier.

Waddell, L. & Taylor, M. (2008). A new self-rating scale for detecting atypical or second-generation antipsychotic side effects. *Journal of Psychopharmacology, 22*(3): 238–243.

World Health Organization (WHO). (2012). *Role of anticholinergic medications in patients requiring long-term antipsychotic treatment for psychotic disorders.* Online. Available: www.who.int/mental_health/mhgap/evidence/resource/psychosis_q6.pdf 11 November 2020.

Yilmaz, D., Khorshid, L., & Dedeoƒülu, Y. (2016). The effect of the Z-track technique on pain and drug leakage in intramuscular injection. *Clinical Nurse Specialist, 30*(6), E7–E12.

WEB RESOURCES

Liverpool University Neuroleptic Side Effect Rating Scale: LUNSERS: https://innovation.ox.ac.uk/outcome-measures/liverpool-university-neuroleptic-side-effect-rating-scale-lunsers/.

National Institute of Mental Health —Mental health medications: www.nimh.nih. gov.health/topics/mental-health-medications/index.shmtl.

National Prescribing Authority (Australia): www.nps.org.au.

Royal Australian College of General Practitioners. (2019). *Polypharmacy in RACGP aged care clinical guide (Silver Book).* Online. Available: www.racgp.org.au/clinical resources/clinical-guidelines/key-racgp-guidelines/view-all-racgp-guidelines/ silver-book/part-a/polypharmacy 26 Nov 2020.

Transcultural Mental Health Centre– Consumer medication brochures: www. dhi.health.nsw.gov.au/transcultural-mental-health-centre-tmhc/resources/ multilingual-resources-by-title/consumer-medication-brochures.

10 CULTURE AND MENTAL HEALTH

INTRODUCTION

In this chapter, the social construct of culture is defined and ways of engaging with people who have mental illness or mental health problems, which take into account the person's cultural background, are examined. The New Zealand model of 'cultural safety' is presented as an exemplar of how mental health professionals can practise in ways that demonstrate cultural competence and how mental health services can provide a culturally inclusive environment in which mental healthcare and treatment can be delivered. Practical examples of culturally competent practice and culturally inclusive environments are also included.

WHAT IS CULTURE?

Culture is a socially defined, dynamic and ever-changing phenomenon that refers to the history, beliefs, language, practices, dress and customs that are shared by a group of people, and that influences the identity, behaviour and values of the members. There is a caveat on this definition, though, because it cannot be assumed that all members of one culture necessarily share identical worldviews on any or all issues. This is particularly so for second-generation immigrants who move between their culture of origin at home and the adopted culture in which they live. Consider, for example, a young person who was born in New Zealand to Vietnamese parents who immigrated in the 1980s. The young person moves between the Vietnamese culture at home and the wider New Zealand culture outside the home. Consequently, the person's cultural practices will be influenced by the context and environment in which they occur.

Commonly, culture is equated with ethnicity, but this is a limited interpretation. Other cultural groupings also exist based on social demographics such as employment, religion or lifestyle. Box 10.1 lists examples of social groups that are united by shared understandings that influence worldview, norms and social interactions.

> **Box 10.1** **Examples of social groups united by shared understandings**
>
> Cultural groups can be defined by:
>
> - ethnicity (a common shared view about ancestry)
> - race (biologically determined by genetic inheritance)
> - sex (however the person identifies)
> - gender (cultural understandings of masculinity and femininity)
> - sexual orientation (gay, lesbian, bisexual, heterosexual)
> - life-span phase (infancy, old age)
> - religion and spirituality (organised/informal)
> - geographical location (metropolitan, regional, remote)
> - socioeconomic status.

Being a member of a cultural group doesn't in itself pose mental health risks. However, if membership of a group leads to social exclusion or stigma based on the person's cultural identity, then negative mental health outcomes may result. For example, lesbian, gay, bisexual, trans, intersex and queer (LGBTIQ) people who experience stigma, prejudice, discrimination and abuse on the grounds of being LGBTIQ Aboriginal are five times more likely to attempt suicide than the general population and twice as likely to be diagnosed with a mental health disorder. The incidence for suicide attempt by transgender people is 11 times that of the general population (National LGBTI Health Alliance 2020).

CULTURE AND RISK OF MENTAL ILLNESS

Some people, as a consequence of their cultural heritage and history, are at increased risk of being diagnosed with a mental illness. Colonisation, for example, has had a devastating effect on the health of the Indigenous peoples of Australia and New Zealand. Similarly, in the US, American Indians, and peoples of the First Nations and Inuit communities in Canada also face a unique set of mental health challenges. At particular risk are people from backgrounds that are culturally and linguistically diverse (CALD) from the mainstream dominant culture, including immigrants, refugees and Indigenous peoples. The diversity of CALD people may also overlap with other 'at risk' population groups such as

---

Box 10.2 **Risk factors for diagnosis of mental illness**

- Previous experience of trauma or flight
- Experience of racism or discrimination
- High levels of stress as a result of integrating into a new culture
- Cultural bereavement or dislocation from community
- Experience of institutional racism and lack of cultural competence within the health system
- Change of traditional roles within the family, and lack of social and family support networks
- Loss of status (e.g. employment, income, role)
- Loss of self-esteem, feelings of powerlessness and communication difficulties
- Lack of access to health and support services
- Language barriers
- Subject of discriminatory behaviour from others

Source: Life in Mind 2021

---

older adults, LGBTI, young people, and rural and remote communities. Factors that have been identified as increasing a person's risk for mental illness can be found in Box 10.2.

EXPLANATORY MODELS OF MENTAL ILLNESS

It is important to recognise that, in the main, theories of mental illness were developed in the Western world but that different interpretations of health and explanations for mental illness exist between cultures and so cultural interpretations of mental illness will vary across the world.

Western medicine, with its individualistic view of health, ascribes responsibility for health to the individual, whereas collectivist cultures emphasise the role of family and community. For example, while recognising the diversity of culture that exists between Aboriginal and Torres Strait Islander people, health and particularly mental health is largely understood within the context of a community. Health is holistic and embedded through connections with kinship, country, land, spirits and ancestors, mind and the body (Australian Indigenous HealthInfoNet 2021). Similarly, traditional Māori beliefs regard health as being influenced by the four domains of mind, spirit, family (extended) and the physical world (Ministry of Health 2017). Consequently, caution must be exercised when applying theories from Western medicine, which are derived from research conducted in individualist societies, to people from collectivist societies such as Australian Aboriginal or Torres Strait Islander peoples, New Zealand Māori, immigrants and refugees. Also, in practice, this may mean that decisions about mental healthcare and treatment for a person whose culture is collective will be made by the extended family and not by the individual, as is the practice in Western individualised cultures.

Furthermore, in some cultures, illness, including mental illness, is usually attributed to external forces or spiritual reasons. This, therefore, makes the Western model of attributing mental illness to an internal disease process inappropriate or irrelevant to their beliefs. In some Asian cultures, value is placed on a person's achievements and emotional self-control, hence experiencing mental illness can bring shame to the family. Similarly, within the Indian culture, the social and hierarchical status of a person is of paramount importance and any issue that has an impact on this, including mental health, is seen as a burden. It is not uncommon for relatives to send the person experiencing mental illness away from the family or as is the case for some people in Indonesia, be confined via shackles, stocks or other restraint mechanisms within the family property due to beliefs of demon possession or bad spirits (Hidayat et al 2020). Additionally, culture can affect the interpretation of voice hearing. In Western medicine, voice hearing is labelled as a hallucination, i.e. a symptom of pathology, whereas in other cultures hearing the voice of a deceased loved one, is a common and spiritual experience. This highlights the importance of cultural context when assessing people who are thought to be experiencing mental illness. What may be considered as 'abnormal' in one culture is acceptable in another. The key is to implement the mental state examination in a manner that is culturally safe, respecting different values and beliefs, while assessing for recent or ongoing changes in behaviour and daily functioning that may support a deterioration of mental health.

THE IMPACT OF CULTURE AND MENTAL HEALTH

Every person is unique. Their experience of mental illness and their road to recovery will likewise be unique. Understanding the role culture plays for individuals and the impact culture can have on a person's health, experience and treatment can help address the inequity of mental healthcare practice and support better health outcomes. It has already been established that people with mental illness face social stigma by the very nature of experiencing a mental health issue. This stigma can be perpetuated by cultural stigma.

Each culture will have a different way of understanding mental illness. For some this can result in a reluctance to speak out or access help for their illness in the fear they will be ostracised from family or community. For others it may be difficult to understand they are experiencing mental health problems since emotional problems are not recognised as a valid health concern. Cultural factors thus determine the level of support offered from family, friends and communities and what resources are accessed. Minority populations are less likely to seek help for their mental health and may only come to the attention of a health service when the symptoms are so severe there is no alternative. Alongside cultural factors, other disparities such as low socioeconomic status, financial burden, homelessness, discrimination and lack of mental health awareness can increase the level of disenfranchisement that is seen in many minority groups.

CULTURAL COMPETENCE

Cultural competence refers to the actions of a provider or health professional. Culturally competent health professionals possess a set of qualities that enable them to deliver care in a culturally respectful manner. They possess the attributes outlined in Box 10.3.

Box 10.3 **Cultural competence: required values of health professionals**

A culturally competent health professional is:

- aware of, respects and accepts difference, including
  - an awareness of their own ancestral history
  - an awareness of their own values and what shapes them
  - a non-judgmental attitude (difference is neither right nor wrong)
  - an ability to treat others with respect
- flexible and responsive to the unexpected
- willing to learn and undertake continuing professional development
- willing to work with ambiguity
- able to manage the dynamics of difference
- confident in working with people from CALD backgrounds
- able to be an advocate with or on behalf of people in their care.

Source: Australian Institute of Health and Welfare 2015

CULTURAL SAFETY

Cultural safety moves beyond cultural competence by focusing on the experience of the person who is the recipient of delivered care. It is more than acknowledging and respecting difference and being sensitive to a person's culture. It recognises the inherent power imbalances and inequity across cultures and seeks to address these through education, health professional accreditations standards, legislation and policy directives. Williams (2008) defines cultural safety as:

> ... an environment, which is safe for people; where there is no assault, challenge or denial of their identity, of who they are and what they need. It is about shared respect, shared meaning, shared knowledge and experience, of learning together with dignity and truly listening.

Cultural safety is a concept derived from the discipline of nursing in New Zealand in the late 1980s in response to recruitment and retention issues regarding Māori nurses and the poor health status of New Zealand's Indigenous people. The model integrates cultural safety with the Treaty of Waitangi and Māori health. Previously, professional codes of ethics directed health professionals to care for people *regardless* of their sex, race, culture, educational or religious backgrounds, whereas the New Zealand cultural safety model directs nurses to *take regard* of these by acknowledging and responding to difference, and to 'take into account all that makes [human beings] unique' (Nursing Council of New Zealand / Te Kaunihera Tapuhi o Aotearoa 2011, p. 7).

Now applicable across all health professionals, the New Zealand model comprises three phases of preparation for culturally safe practice (see Table 10.1). First, *cultural awareness* sensitises students and health professionals to their own cultural heritage and to difference. This is followed by *cultural sensitivity*, which alerts students and health

TABLE 10.1
Phases of preparation for culturally safe healthcare practice

Phase	Description
Cultural awareness	Awareness of difference and own cultural heritage
Cultural sensitivity	Acceptance of the legitimacy of difference
Cultural safety	Occurs when the person perceives healthcare to be delivered in a manner that preserves and respects cultural heritage

Source: Nursing Council of New Zealand/Te Kaunihera Tapuhi o Aotearoa 2011

professionals to the legitimacy of difference. Finally, *cultural safety* is achieved when the person perceives that the healthcare was delivered in a manner that respected and preserved their cultural integrity. This is an important feature of the New Zealand model (i.e. that cultural safety is identified by the person receiving care, not the health professional providing care). It is the person who determines whether or not they have been cared for in a culturally appropriate (safe) way. Finally, the model requires not only that health professionals be culturally competent but also that health services provide a culturally inclusive environment.

A culturally inclusive environment

A culturally inclusive environment is one in which the organisation has structures in place to ensure difference is respected, discrimination is not tolerated and the special needs of people from CALD backgrounds are accommodated. It possesses the attributes outlined in Box 10.4.

CULTURAL AND LINGUISTIC DIVERSITY

Across the world's people there are over 7000 languages spoken. The world is full of different people with different cultures, traditions and

---

Box 10.4 Features of a culturally inclusive environment

A culturally inclusive environment is one in which:

- difference is acknowledged, valued and respected
- difference is accommodated (i.e. the organisation is structured to respond to individual needs such as access to interpreters and gender-appropriate health professionals)
- policies are in place to protect people in care (e.g. equal opportunity) and these policies are followed, including consequences if they are not
- cultural knowledge is institutionalised in policy and practice
- cultural self-assessments are conducted
- people with mental illness and staff feel free to
  - express their cultural identity
  - express their opinions and values
  - engage in cultural practices (e.g. prayer)
  - feel safe from unfair criticism, abuse or harassment.

Source: Australian Institute of Health and Welfare 2015

customs. Increased possibilities of travel have allowed opportunity for people to visit and live in places once never thought possible. Countries now have expanding populations and increasing cultural and linguistic diversity as people move around the globe. For example, for more than 200 years, immigration has expanded the populations of Australia and New Zealand and thereby contributed to the diverse ethnic cultural makeup of these two nations. Within these two countries, 3.3% identify themselves as Indigenous Australians (Australian Institute of Health and Welfare 2019), and 16.7% identify as Māori (Statistics New Zealand 2018) with the rest of the demographic population established from colonisation and the extensive migration of diverse cultures. This has developed a rich and varied use of language spoken within the home. It is clearly evident that multiculturalism and cultural diversity are defining features around the world and therefore cultural awareness in the health sector is key to providing equitable healthcare and recognising disparities, particularly for a number of people who have been discriminated against based on their ethnic origin, skin colour, sexuality or religion.

Working with interpreters

When English is not the person's first language or a cultural consultant is required, an interpreter can facilitate communication and understanding (including verbal, non-verbal and written). This applies to Indigenous peoples as well as people from a CALD background. When available, always use a professionally trained interpreter, either in person, via a telephone interpreter service or via a teleconference. Avoid using family members or ancillary or other staff members, except in an emergency. They may have a conflict of interest or may not be able to accurately translate medical or psychiatric terminology, and the person may withhold information because of their relationship with the person. See Box 10.5 (overleaf) for guidelines regarding working with an interpreter.

Working with people from an Indigenous or CALD background

When working with people from an Indigenous or CALD background it is important to be prepared. Use the information in Box 10.3 and Box 10.4 to reflect on your own cultural competence and to assess how culturally inclusive your workplace is. Additionally, you can prepare yourself by undertaking training courses (e.g. a 'cross-cultural competency' or a 'working with an interpreter' course) and by becoming familiar with the Indigenous and multicultural services in your organisation and within the community. These services and agencies can assist communication and understanding. Importantly, avoid using stereotypes, be flexible in your approach,

Box 10.5	Guidelines for conducting an interview with an interpreter

Pre-interview

- Always use a professionally trained interpreter, except in an emergency.
- Be prepared. Have the contact details of the interpreter service and telephone interpreter service on the health unit's list of frequently used numbers.
- If possible, book the interpreter well in advance to ensure the availability of the most suitable interpreter.
- Match the person and interpreter as closely as possible. Seek more than a language match. Consider also ethnicity, religion, migration history and political context.
- Avoid using family members or ancillary or other staff members, except in an emergency.
- Consider whether the interpreter needs to be a specific gender. Ask the person with mental illness about gender preference.
- Check whether the interpreter and the person know each other socially or have a relationship.
- Optimise seating and other spatial arrangements.
- Set a time for a pre-brief and post-interview discussion with the interpreter.
- Consider safety. Identify a code word to use if the meeting needs to be stopped.

During the interview

- Introduce everyone and their role.
- Explain the purpose of the interview.
- Explain that confidentiality will be observed.
- Explain that the interpreter and the health professional may take notes during the interview.
- Explain that everything will be translated.
- Ensure that only one person speaks at a time.
- Address questions to the person, not the interpreter. Speak to the person in the first person.
- Look at the person when the interpreter is reporting the person's response.
- Avoid using technical language, jargon or slang.

- Use short sentences and pause frequently to enable the interpreter to translate.

Post-interview

- Have a debrief discussion with the interpreter.
- Give and seek feedback on how the interview went.
- Ask the interpreter for their comments and concerns.
- Identify safety issues.

Source: Australian Psychological Society 2013; Victorian Transcultural Mental Health 2019.

demonstrate a willingness to learn and be open to the fact that the person's view of health may differ from your own and/or the mainstream view.

Nevertheless, while a cultural safety model directs health professionals to seek understanding of difference, and to accept and work with difference, such acceptance must not be undertaken in the absence of critique. Some practices, which are purported to be cultural, can transgress the values and laws of the wider society. For example, customs like denying education to girls, or sexual relationships between adults and children, must be challenged, rather than accepted without being questioned.

CASE STUDY

New Zealand Māori

Traditional Māori views of health acknowledge the link between the mind, the spirit, the connection with family (whānau) and the physical world in a way that is seamless and natural. Until the introduction of Western medicine, there was no division between these four domains. Consequently, Māori philosophy towards health is based on a wellness (holistic health) model in which whānau (family health), tinana (physical health), hinengaro (mental health) and wairua (spiritual health) comprise the four cornerstones (or sides) of Māori health. Many Māori believe the major deficiency in modern health services is in taha wairua (the spiritual dimension).

Māori view mental health as the capacity to think and to feel that mind and body are interconnected and one, and therefore inseparable. Thoughts, feelings and emotions are integral components of the body and soul. This is how Māori see themselves in the universe, how they interact with that which is uniquely Māori, and the perceptions that others have of Māori (Russell 2018).

Indigenous Australians

Generally, Australian Indigenous culture is holistic; therefore, concepts of mental illness must 'take into account the entirety of one's experiences, including physical, mental, emotional, spiritual and obviously cultural states of being'. Indigenous Australians attribute illness to external events, which are likely to be culturally based, with mental illness viewed as a sickness of spirit, heart and mind. Common attributions for illness, including mental illness, are 'doing something wrong culturally' or 'being paid back' for wrongdoing. This reflects the intertwining of spirituality and, particularly, relationships with family, land and culture.

(Korff 2021)

CONCLUSION

Like healthcare in general, culturally safe mental healthcare is based on social justice and equity principles that advocate the importance of knowledge acquisition, mutual respect and negotiation. This chapter has outlined strategies that facilitate culturally safe mental healthcare and has presented the New Zealand model of cultural safety as a framework for providing culturally appropriate care and treatment in mental health settings. The model proposes that for health services to be culturally safe, they need to be provided in an environment that is culturally inclusive and delivered by health professionals who are culturally competent. The model is equally applicable in mental health contexts as it is in general health settings.

REFERENCES

Australian Indigenous HealthInfoNet. (2021). *Summary of Aboriginal and Torres Strait Islander health status—selected topics 2020.* Perth: Australian Indigenous HealthInfoNet. Online. Available: https://healthinfonet.ecu.edu.au/learn/health-facts/summary-aboriginal-torres-strait-islander-health/42693/?title=Summary%20 of%20Aboriginal%20and%20Torres%20Strait%20Islander%20health%20 status%20-%20selected%20topics%202020&contentid=42693_21 April 2021.

Australian Institute of Health and Welfare. (2015). *Cultural competency in the delivery of health services for Indigenous people,* Closing the Gap Clearinghouse, Issue paper no. 13. Online. Available: https://www.aihw.gov.au/reports/indigenous-australians/cultural-competency-in-the-delivery-of-health-services-for-indigenous-people/contents/table-of-contents 19 March 2021.

Australian Institute of Health and Welfare. (2019). *Profile of Indigenous Australians.* Online. Available: https://www.aihw.gov.au/reports/australias-welfare/profile-of-indigenous-australians 13 May 2021.

Australian Psychological Society. (2013). *Working with interpreters: a practice guide for psychologists.* Melbourne: APS. Online. Available: https://ausit.org/wp-content/uploads/2020/02/APS-Working-with-Interpreters-Practice-Guide-for-Psychologists_2013.pdf 19 March 2021.

Hidayat, M.T., Lawn, S., Muir-Cochrane, E. et al. (2020). The use of pasung for people with mental illness: a systematic review and narrative synthesis. *International Journal of Mental Health Systems, 14*, 90.

Korff, J. 2021. *Mental health and Aboriginal people.* Online. Available: https://www.creativespirits.info/aboriginalculture/health/mental-health-and-aboriginal-people 20th March 2021.

Life in Mind. (2021). *Culturally and linguistically diverse communities.* Online. Available: https://lifeinmind.org.au/about-suicide/other-population-groups/culturally-and-linguistically-diverse-communities 19 March 2021.

Ministry of Health. (2017). *Māori health models.* Online. Available: https://www.health.govt.nz/our-work/populations/maori-health/maori-health-models/maori-health-models-te-whare-tapa-wha 18 March 2021.

National LGBTI Health Alliance. (2020). *Snapshot of mental health and suicide prevention statistics for LGBTI people.* Online. Available: https://d3n8a8pro7vhmx.cloudfront.net/lgbtihealth/pages/549/attachments/original/1595492235/2020-Snapshot_mental_health_%281%29.pdf?1595492235 17 March 2021.

Nursing Council of New Zealand / Te Kaunihera Tapuhi o Aotearoa. (2011). *Guidelines for cultural safety, the Treaty of Waitangi and Māori health in nursing education and practice* (2nd ed.). Wellington: NCNZ. Online. Available: http://ndhadeliver.natlib.govt.nz/delivery/DeliveryManagerServlet?dps_pid=IE6429026&dps_custom_att_1=ilsdbviewed 19 March 2021.

Statistics New Zealand. (2018). *2018 Census.* Online. Available: https://www.stats.govt.nz/tools/2018-census-place-summaries/new-zealand#ethnicity-culture-and-identity 17 March 2021.

Russell, L. (2018). Te Oranga Hinengaro: Report on *Māori* mental wellbeing results from the New Zealand Mental Health Monitor & Health and Lifestyles Survey. Wellington: Health Promotion Agency/Te Hiringa Hauora.

Victorian Transcultural Mental Health. (2019). *Approaching work with interpreters in mental health settings.* Online. Available: https://vtmh.org.au/wpcontent/uploads/2008/01/VTMHProjectreport.pdf 20th March 2021.

Williams, R. (2008) Cultural safety: what does it mean for our work practice? *Australian and New Zealand Journal of Public Health, 23*(2), 213–214.

WEB RESOURCES

Australian Indigenous Healthinfonet: www.healthinfonet.ecu.edu.au. This site provides comprehensive and up-to-date information for anyone interested in the health of Indigenous Australians. It aims to contribute to 'closing the gap' in health between Indigenous and non-Indigenous Australians by informing practice and policy in Indigenous health by making research and other knowledge readily accessible.

Embrace Multicultural Mental Health: www.embracementalhealth.org.au A site where resources, information and services can be found for people from culturally and linguistically diverse backgrounds.

Māori Health: www.maorihealth.govt.nz. This site provides information about Māori health and highlights the policies, programs and people who are addressing Māori health.

Multicultural Mental Health Australia: www.mmha.org.au. Multicultural Mental Health Australia provides national leadership in building greater awareness of mental health and suicide prevention among Australians from CALD backgrounds.

Victorian Transcultural Mental Health: www.vtmh.org.au. The VTMH is a statewide unit that supports area mental health and psychiatric disability support services in working with CALD people and carers throughout Victoria.

11 CO-OCCURRING MEDICAL PROBLEMS

INTRODUCTION

This chapter explores common medical problems that co-exist in people with mental illness. All health professionals and workers in social services and residential support settings will encounter people with physical conditions who also have a mental health problem. Health professionals, including general practitioners, physiotherapists, occupational therapists and nurses are well placed to provide holistic care for both physical and mental healthcare needs and therefore to screen and develop a management plan for people with physical health problems. While the physical health needs of people with mental illness is now receiving more attention, recent research identified physical health as a neglected area of care in mental health services (Gray & Brown 2017).

THE EXTENT OF THE PROBLEM

Experiencing mental illness is often linked to poorer health outcomes, higher rates of disability, comorbidity and increased mortality. For example, in comparison to those without a mental illness, individuals with a severe mental disorder are at far greater risk of cardiovascular and metabolic diseases (Firth et al 2019) and have a two to three times higher average of dying prematurely than the general population, owing to physical health problems that are often not treated, such as cancers, cardiovascular diseases, respiratory disease, diabetes and HIV infection (WHO 2018). Although the rate of death due to heart disease has decreased in the general population over the past 20 years, this has not occurred in people with an enduring mental illness. The need to recognise the physical needs of people with a broad range of mental illnesses has been emphasised worldwide particularly in populations such as in low- to middle-income countries where the global burden of disease from mental illness appears to be increasing. Behaviours including smoking, lack of exercise, poor self-care and poor diet have all been identified as contributing factors that lead to these poor health outcomes.

The following health conditions are common to people living with enduring mental illness, who are much more likely to experience such conditions compared with the rest of the population.

- Gum disease and loss of teeth
- Respiratory disease
- Diabetes
- Sexual dysfunction
- Hyperlipidaemia (high levels of lipids (fats) in the bloodstream)
- Cardiovascular disease including hypertension and cardiac arrhythmias
- Gastrointestinal disorders and bowel cancer

There is some evidence that people seriously affected by symptoms of severe or enduring mental illness have a different perception of pain. While some report a higher pain threshold and a diminished response to pain, in contrast others experience pain more frequently with stronger intensity. Reasons for this are speculative, though common features identified appear dependent on the symptoms of mental illness being experienced (den Boer et al 2019). Ultimately, health professionals need to have a heightened awareness of such issues so they are able to meet the somatic needs of people with a lived experience of mental illness and deliver optimum care.

Obesity continues to be a significant health condition for people with mental illness. Both lifestyle factors such as poor diet and lack of exercise (Taylor et al 2020) and features of illness such as lack of motivation and poor energy levels increase weight gain. Without early intervention, when a person commences taking antipsychotics, they are invariably going to gain weight. Clozapine and olanzapine are strongly associated with weight gain, but a number of other antipsychotics are also responsible (Marteene et al 2019). Obesity can also have an impact on a person's mental health. People who are severely overweight are four times more likely to experience depressive symptoms than people without a significant weight problem. This linear relationship between mental illness and obesity does not only occur in adults. It has also been identified in children and young people so that if one occurs, it increases the chance of the other occurring. Not surprisingly, the comorbidity of obesity and severe mental illness can lead to adverse health outcomes such as poor quality of life, and an increase in the physical health mortality and morbidity rate in comparison to that of the general population. Metabolic syndrome and diabetes mellitus (discussed later in the chapter) are strongly associated with mental illnesses due to the serious side effect of obesity from the antipsychotic medications prescribed. Obesity, cigarette smoking and alcohol and substance abuse are all significant health risks for people with enduring mental illnesses such as schizophrenia, depression and bipolar affective disorder. These issues place people with mental illness as a significantly vulnerable group, with associated social, economic and health burdens on society as a whole (WHO 2018).

Those working with people with mental health problems can facilitate optimal health by enquiring about physical health complaints as well as use of alcohol, tobacco and illicit substances. Encouraging and assisting people to access health services and have health check-ups can reduce the long-term damaging effects of such behaviours. Primary healthcare workers are ideally positioned to screen for high blood pressure, respiratory problems, diabetes and metabolic syndrome.

METABOLIC SYNDROME

Metabolic syndrome can be defined as a cluster of risk factors for obesity, insulin resistance and cardiovascular disease. People with a mental illness such as schizophrenia and bipolar disorder have an increased prevalence of metabolic syndrome and its associated conditions such as high blood pressure, high blood glucose levels, high levels of triglycerides, low HDL levels (good cholesterol) and excess body fat around the waist. Often associated with antipsychotic medications, the presence of metabolic syndrome can be detected through medical history taking, anthropometry (body mass index (see Box 11.1) and hip/waist

---

Box 11.1   Body Mass Index

BMI is determined by a person's weight in kilograms divided by their height in metres squared. The formula is:

$$BMI = \frac{Weight\,(kg)}{Height\,(m)^2}$$

The BMI is designed for men and women over the age of 18. A healthy BMI is between 20 and 25. A result below 20 indicates that the person may be underweight, while a result above 25 indicates that the person may be overweight. A BMI over 30 indicates a risk of developing metabolic syndrome. The BMI is of limited use across populations who may be much smaller in height or heavier in weight than Caucasians but is an easy tool to use in the first instance.

Girth measurement (the measurement around the waist) is a basic indicator of risk of heart disease, with men at risk above 102 cm and women above 88 cm.

Box 11.2   **Diagnostic criteria for metabolic syndrome**

Diagnostic criteria include:

- a waist circumference > 94 cm for men and > 80 cm for women
- BMI over 30
- raised blood triglyceride and raised cholesterol levels (measured through blood tests)
- raised blood pressure (BP): systolic BP > 130 mmHg or diastolic BP > 85 mmHg (or treatment for hypertension in the past)
- raised fasting plasma glucose > 5.6 mmol/L (or previously diagnosed type 2 diabetes).

---

circumference), blood pressure measurement and measurement of lipid values and blood or plasma glucose. Box 11.2 lists the diagnostic criteria for metabolic syndrome.

DIABETES MELLITUS

Metabolic syndrome and diabetes mellitus are intricately connected due to the increased risk of diabetes type 2 in people with a metabolic disorder. Similarly, both are closely connected as a major health concern for people with a mental illness. As already established, this can be related to the use of antipsychotic medication (Hirsch et al 2018), however other factors must also be taken into consideration such as lack of physical exercise and poor diet which can exacerbate the risk of diabetes. It is also well established that people with diabetes are far more likely to experience mental health issues such as anxiety and depression, which, in turn, can impact on daily self-management. Such problems often go undiagnosed and thus untreated since health professionals may explain behaviour and mood changes as diabetes distress which is a common emotional response to living with diabetes.

Screening of people for depression, anxiety and diabetes alongside regular monitoring of blood, including glucose helps identify problems early to allow appropriate interventions to be implemented.

PREVENTION AND MANAGEMENT: ONGOING MONITORING

Ongoing physical monitoring of the person is important, as regular monitoring of basic observations can greatly assist the early recognition, prevention and management of chronic health issues. Health professionals can carry out basic observations such as:

- weight, including BMI
- BP, temperature, respirations
- oral care (teeth, lips, gums)
- skin care, rashes, infections
- foot care, including nails.

FACTORS AFFECTING POOR PHYSICAL HEALTH

There are many factors that contribute to a person having poor overall health. Having a mental illness can negatively affect a person's physical health in a variety of ways. People with mental illness may experience symptoms such as suspicious thoughts, paranoia, depression or poor motivation, making them less likely to leave their homes to go for a walk or plan shopping trips or socialising. They are more likely to make short local trips and buy food that requires little preparation because of their reduced cognitive ability and associated lack of motivation. Physical symptoms from co-occurring illnesses such as pain, reduced mobility and respiratory problems can further reduce physical activity and increase social isolation.

Healthy foods are often expensive in comparison with ready-made frozen foods or fast foods, and people with mental illness are likely to be on low incomes, compounding their health risks. A diet low in fibre, vegetables and fruit, and little physical exercise, increases the likelihood of cardiovascular disease, high blood pressure and stroke (Teasdale et al 2019). Hence, an interplay between behaviours such as smoking, alcohol and substance abuse, combined with symptoms of mental and physical illness, create health problems and poor quality of life for those people living with mental illness. For a number of reasons, people with mental illness do not always receive adequate physical healthcare. These can include diagnostic overshadowing, a lack of an integrated health service and inaccurate self-assessment of symptoms with poor reporting of physical symptoms by people with mental illness.

STRATEGIES FOR IMPROVING PHYSICAL HEALTH

Exercise is an effective strategy for improving general physical and emotional health. Walking is the easiest activity for encouraging people with mental illness to exercise. Engaging people in community walking groups can increase exercise and also provides opportunities for socialisation. Reducing cigarette smoking (by connecting people with national 'Quit' programs) is also an important lifestyle change, together with attention to a healthy diet. Reminding people about the availability of free health checks and providing information about community health centres can also be useful.

It is vital that health professionals engage with people with mental illness about practical ways to increase their physical health and assist them to develop plans for self-care management of their mental health. Referral to an exercise physiologist is a useful mechanism to support the person's physical and mental health. Other strategies include encouraging annual medical and dental check-ups, including full blood tests and electrocardiograms, and providing brochures about prostate checks, mammograms, cervical smear (pap) tests and bone density tests for people older than 50. Encouraging people to attend their closest general practice clinic and to visit them on a regular basis can facilitate an effective working relationship and allow for early recognition of symptoms.

A primary care focus

People with mental health problems often have physical health needs that are not being adequately screened for and treated and are routinely overlooked (Firth et al 2019, Morgan et al 2017). Health professionals can promote health by addressing both the physical and mental health needs of people rather than focusing on one specific disease or health issue. Providing education and training to support staff in the early identification, management and ongoing care strategies will go a long way to improve global health outcomes (Cohen 2017).

Population-targeted strategies including lifestyle, nutrition, exercise, education and improved access to services can reduce health outcomes. Primary care professionals, particularly the GP, are well positioned to address the modifiable factors that contribute to physical comorbidity in people with mental illness. Establishing partnerships and coordinating care with a person, service providers, and family and carers can assist to monitor health and manage emerging physical health conditions by regular screening and implementing early interventions that will promote health and prevent the onset of chronic health conditions. It is just as important to remember that mental illness can occur at any age and for health professionals to not focus purely on an older population. Young people are at high risk of physical illnesses too and hence need a clearly identified approach to support them in maintaining their health. Similarly, the high burden of physical health problems among various populations such as Indigenous peoples and those in developing countries require health promotion initiatives and early intervention as part of a responsive strategy to ensure an integrated approach to health (see Figure 11.1).

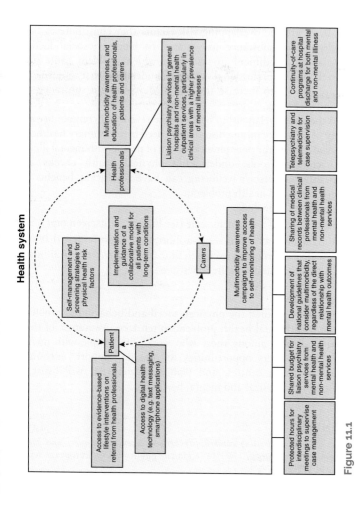

Figure 11.1
Proposed model of collaborative care for people with physical and mental comorbidities
Firth et al 2019

COMORBIDITY AND SUBSTANCE USE

Comorbidity between mental and substance misuse disorders is also common globally. People with a substance misuse disorder have high comorbid rates of mental disorders. Substances include alcohol, tobacco, marijuana and other illicit substances such as methamphetamine and cocaine. There are the overlapping risk factors that contribute to both mental illness and substance use related to biopsychosocial factors; therefore, it can be difficult to ascertain which problem came first. Central to the health professional's role is to understand that some mental illnesses are known to increase the risk of developing a substance use disorder and vice versa.

Due to the strong relationship between the severity of comorbidity and the severity of substance misuse disorders we need better primary healthcare approaches to address the poor physical health of people with mental illness.

Using screening tools, undertaking physical health checks and enquiring about a person's wellbeing can have significant benefits for people with comorbid health problems.

Assessment scales include:

- the AUDIT alcohol assessment scale (see https://auditscreen.org/)
- the CAGE alcohol screening test—a short, four-question test that diagnoses alcohol problems over a lifetime (see https://www.healthline.com/health/cage-questionnaire#questions).

CONCLUSION

This chapter has explored the physical, social and behavioural problems that people with mental health problems often face. Awareness of these additional challenges among those who work with people with mental health problems offers opportunities to provide support, encourage attendance at health centres, and plan strategies that will assist in maintaining both physical and mental health.

REFERENCES

Cohen, A. (2017). *Addressing comorbidity between mental disorders and major noncommunicable diseases.* WHO regional publications. European series. Denmark: WHO.

den Boer, K., de Veer, A.J.E., Schoonmade, L.J. et al. (2019) A systematic review of palliative care tools and interventions for people with severe mental illness. *BMC Psychiatry, 19*, 106.

Firth, J., Siddiqi, N., Koyanagi, A., et al. (2019). The Lancet Psychiatry Commission: a blueprint for protecting physical health in people with mental illness. *The Lancet Psychiatry, 6*(8), 675–712.

Gray, R., & Brown, E. (2017). What does mental health nursing contribute to improving the physical health of service users with severe mental illness? A thematic analysis. *International Journal of Mental Health Nursing, 26*(1), 32–40.

Hirsch, L., Patten, S.B., Bresee, L., et al. (2018). Second-generation antipsychotics and metabolic side-effects: Canadian population-based study. *British Journal of Psychiatry Open, 4*(4), 256–261.

Marteene, W., Winckel, K., Hollingworth, S., et al. (2019) Strategies to counter antipsychotic-associated weight gain in patients with schizophrenia. *Expert Opinion on Drug Safety, 18*(12), 1150–1160.

Morgan, V.A., Waterreus, A., Carr, V., et al. (2017). Responding to challenges for people with psychotic illness: updated evidence from the Survey of High Impact Psychosis. *Australian and New Zealand Journal of Psychiatry, 51*(2), 124–140.

Taylor, V.H., Sockalingam, S., Hawa, R., & Hahn, M. (2020) Canadian adult obesity clinical practice guidelines: the role of mental health in obesity management. Online. Available: https://obesitycanada.ca/guidelines/mentalhealth 8 November 2020.

Teasdale, S., Ward, P., Samaras, K., et al. (2019). Dietary intake of people with severe mental illness: systematic review and meta-analysis. *The British Journal of Psychiatry, 214*(5), 251–259.

World Health Organization (WHO). (2018). *Guidelines for the management of physical health conditions in adults with severe mental disorders.* Geneva: WHO.

WEB RESOURCES

Comorbidity: substance use and other mental disorders—National Institute on Drug Abuse (NIDA): https://www.drugabuse.gov/drug-topics/trends-statistics/infographics/comorbidity-substance-use-other-mental-disorders. This website provides data and information on substance use and mental health issues in the USA.

Depression and mental health—Diabetes Australia: https://www.diabetesaustralia.com.au/living-with-diabetes/preventing-complications/depression-and-mental-health/. This website offers information to people with diabetes experiencing depression.

Healthy Active Lives (HeAL): www.iphys.org.au. HeAL is a statement that aims to reverse the trend of people with mental illness dying early by addressing risks for future physical illnesses early and proactively.

Mental Health Partnerships: http://mentalhealthpartnerships.com/resource/physical-health-checks-for-people-with-smi/. This is a brief tool that enables health professionals to work with consumers to screen physical health and take evidence-based action when variables are identified to be at risk.

WHO—A guide for tobacco users to quit: https://www.who.int/tobacco/publications/smoking_cessation/9789241506939/en/. This website provides quit smoking assistance, assessment tools and information.

12 LOSS AND GRIEF

INTRODUCTION

Change, transition and loss are constant features of everyday life. Loss can have a major impact on the person involved (e.g. the death of a parent) or it may be less significant (e.g. moving house, losing your wallet). The experience of grief and mourning following a significant loss can be intense, including distressing affective, cognitive and behavioural responses. Nevertheless, as upsetting as they are, such reactions are normal and are not necessarily evidence of a mental health problem.

Health professionals constantly work with people who are experiencing loss and, thereby, may find themselves in the unique position of being a key support person in a significant experience for someone who is grieving. This chapter examines the concept of loss and bereavement and identifies ways that health professionals can understand and best assist a bereaved person. It goes on to help identify when grief and loss may require specialist input due to its severity or enduring nature of presentation.

UNDERSTANDING LOSS, GRIEF AND MOURNING

Loss involves the separation from a person or an object that has meaning to the person and to which the person feels strongly connected (Barkway & Bull 2019). The loss may be tangible (e.g. the death of a loved one) or intangible (e.g. loss of self-esteem following redundancy). The period in which the person experiences grief (affective) reactions and engages in mourning behaviours is referred to as 'bereavement'. Table 12.1 (overleaf) distinguishes between the terms 'loss', 'grief', 'mourning' and 'bereavement'.

While loss and grief experiences are distressing, they are a normal human response and not usually indicative of mental illness. People of all ages grieve. Rather than accept death and grief as a normal part of life, some cultures have developed strategies to protect people, particularly

TABLE 12.1
Loss, grief, mourning and bereavement

Term	Definition
Loss	Being parted from someone or something that the person values
Grief	The affective (emotional) component of mourning, including the painful affects (feelings) associated with the loss (e.g. sadness, anger, guilt, shame, anxiety)
Mourning	The behavioural component of bereavement, which includes biological reactions, behavioural responses and cognitive and defensive reactions related to the loss
Bereavement	The experience of grief and mourning

children, from this intrinsic life event. Not allowing children to say 'goodbye', attend culture-bound death rites, or be witness to others' distress can in turn impact management of their own emotions and ability to develop appropriate psychological coping mechanisms to move though the grieving process. Grief responses are individual and vary with each person—that is, the magnitude of the loss and the meaning the loss has for the bereaved person. Responses can include feelings of deep sadness, anger, guilt and despair; cognitive reactions can include disbelief, confusion and ruminations about the loss. Mourning responses include physical reactions such as fatigue and a hyper-startle response, and behavioural responses like social withdrawal and sleep disturbances. Older adults are more susceptible to physiological changes as a response to grief rather than recognising the illness or physical symptoms they are experiencing as a somatic manifestation associated with their grief and emotions. Some behavioural responses are life enhancing (e.g. crying and talking about the loss) and facilitate grieving, but others are life depleting (e.g. excessive drinking or making suicidal gestures) and potentially harmful for the person.

Mourning responses are culturally determined. For example, traditional Indigenous cultures often have more prescribed mourning practices than those found in Anglo-European Australian or New Zealand cultures. Tangihanga, the Māori approach to the process of grieving, includes protocols and practices to not only mourn the person who has died but also the ancestors who have passed before them (Mead 2016).

MODELS AND THEORIES OF LOSS AND BEREAVEMENT

Models and theories of loss and bereavement in order to understand and thereby assist the bereaved have been proposed since the middle of the 20th century. Kübler-Ross's influential model identified the phases a dying person experiences as they approach their death. These phases included denial, anger, bargaining, depression and acceptance (Kübler-Ross 1969). Kübler-Ross never intended her model to apply to all losses, and nor did she describe the phases as sequential, though some health professionals have applied the model in this way (Kübler-Ross and Kessler 2014).

Another contemporary model of grieving has been proposed by William Worden (2018). He identifies the tasks of mourning as:

- accept the reality of the loss
- experience the pain of grief
- adjust to the environment where the 'loss' is missing
- emotionally relocate the 'loss' and move on with life.

According to Worden, accomplishing these tasks marks the completion of grieving, though he does not prescribe a period within which this should occur, and nor does he propose that everyone complete this grief experience. Rather, Worden stresses that mourning is a long-term, sometimes lifelong, process. Additionally, Worden states that the completion of grieving does not return the person to their pre-bereavement state—rather, the bereaved person is now able to think about the loss without intense pain and has integrated the experience into their new post-bereavement life.

Finally, while theories and models of loss and mourning provide useful insights into the experience of the bereaved, they must be used cautiously because everyone's loss experience is different. Grieving is not a linear experience, grief has no end point, culture influences grief and mourning responses and loss is not always a negative experience (e.g. when death follows a long period of suffering or disability).

UNCOMPLICATED GRIEF

Grief is the normal affective response to loss. Most people's grief will be uncomplicated. Nevertheless, the person's bereavement experience may be distressing and disrupt their lives in the short term, such as after a natural disaster like an earthquake, or following the death of a loved one. The person's grief may also be upsetting for bystanders (including health professionals), who can feel helpless because they are unable to relieve the person's pain. During this period, the bereaved require support as

---

Box 12.1   Strategies for supporting the grieving person

Supportive strategies include the following.

- Contact the person as soon as you hear of the death and express your sorrow for their loss—give a hug if appropriate.
- Maintain contact by
  - visiting (visits don't have to be lengthy)
  - telephoning, writing or sending a card if you are unable to visit.
- Listen if the person wants to talk about the deceased or tell their story again and again—listening is possibly the most important thing you can do.
- Talk about the person who has died.
- Accept extreme behaviours (e.g. crying, screaming, being quiet, laughing).
- Accept expressions of anger, guilt and blame.
- Indicate that grief takes time.
- Include children in the grieving process.
- Be sensitive about dates that might be upsetting or significant for the bereaved person such as anniversaries, birthdays or Mother's Day.
- Offer practical help such as cooking a meal, child minding or walking the dog.
- Try to understand and accept the person—everyone's grief response is different.

Source: GriefLink 2019c

---

they accept the reality of the loss and adjust to living their life without the person or lost object. Strategies that support people experiencing uncomplicated grief are listed in Box 12.1.

Some strategies, however, are not supportive of grieving and may actually hinder uncomplicated grief. Unhelpful strategies, identified by (Grieflink 2019c), are listed in Box 12.2 (overleaf).

COMPLICATED GRIEF

Complicated grief may affect between 10% and 20% of people who are grieving. It is difficult to distinguish complicated from uncomplicated grief, especially in the first six months, because intense emotional,

Box 12.2	Strategies that may be unhelpful to the grieving person

Unhelpful strategies include:

- avoiding talking about the deceased person
- using platitudes and clichés
- offering false reassurance
- telling the person: 'I know how you feel'
- inhibiting the person's grief experience by offering advice about what they should think, feel or do
- ceasing contact with the person if the going gets 'too heavy'
- advising the person on how to grieve, or trying to explain or rationalise their feelings
- having expectations of how the person should grieve and judging the person by these expectations
- taking over and doing things the person can do for themselves
- making comparisons between the person's and others' losses
- using theories of grief to predict experience
- changing the subject (it dismisses the importance of what the person is saying)
- comparing your losses to the bereaved person's loss
- talking about your own grief experiences (unless the bereaved person finds this relevant to their situation and invites you to tell your story).

Help find meaning in the loss

- Meaning making in grief is highly individual, but health professionals can facilitate the process.
- Ask the griever what their loss has meant to them, and share stories of how others have found meaning.
- Share your own perceptions of meaning (e.g. 'It sounds like your life would never have been as happy without your relationship with ...').
- Introduce the griever to meaning-making exercises (e.g. Neimeyer 2019).

Facilitate emotional relocation of the deceased or lost object

- Support the griever in remembering and reminiscing about who/what has been lost.
- Support the griever regarding concrete efforts to remain connected to the lost person or thing.
- Be cautious about a griever's efforts to quickly find a 'replacement'.

Provide time to grieve

- Recognise that active grieving can take time (one to two years, or longer).
- Avoid giving messages that people should 'be over' their grief.
- Remember and support continuing grief at special times (e.g. on the anniversary of a death, birthdays or holidays).
- Educate the griever's support system (family, friends) that grieving takes time.

Interpret normal behaviour

- Help the griever to understand and 'make sense' of their often intense grief responses.
- Assure the griever that their reactions are not uncommon while still acknowledging how they might be upset or worried about their reactions.
- Connect the griever with those who have had similar experiences (e.g. support groups).

Allow for individual differences

- Recognise the great diversity of grieving responses.
- Avoid imposing a 'prescription' about how grievers should react.
- Educate those around the griever that differences in grieving styles and methods are to be expected.

Consider defences and coping styles

- Watch for potentially unhelpful grief responses such as excessive use of alcohol or drugs, withdrawal, refusal to be reminded of the loss or 'burying' oneself in work or some other activity.
- Within a trusting relationship, help the griever explore more useful ways of coping.

Identify grief complications and refer

- Monitor for grief complications (see 'Complicated grief' in this chapter).
- In keeping with professional ethics, recognise your own practice limitations.
- Refer grievers with complications for more advanced assistance.

Source: Barkway & Bull 2019, adapted from Worden 2018

cognitive and behavioural responses to loss are normal and are observed in both circumstances. Nevertheless, indicators for complicated grief include suicidal thoughts and gestures, depressive disorders, post-traumatic stress reactions and persistent grief reactions. People whose grief is complicated may engage in life-depleting behaviours such as compulsive or excessive actions like overeating, shopping or gambling, or agitated, aggressive and demanding behaviours (Worden 2018).

LOSS AND MENTAL ILLNESS

Medicalising bereavement by including grief reactions as a possible mental health disorder has historically been met with resistance. Due to the very nature of emotional pain being an understandable and appropriate response to death, at what point does normal grieving become a disorder? Concerns have been raised that it may be difficult to differentiate between depression and grief, resulting in an increase in antidepressant prescribing from some primary healthcare professionals. This, in turn, led to older versions of the *Diagnostic and Statistical Manual of Mental Disorders* (DSM) to exclude the diagnosis of first onset major depressive disorder if a bereavement had occurred (within the last six months) unless other symptoms were present. Other concerns related to the difficulty in attaching a uniform medical diagnosis on to something (grief) that manifests differently across cultures. More recently an increased understanding in how mourning can present has meant steps have been taken to acknowledge the different forms of mourning and the grieving process and that many people who experience grief go on to experience prolonged grief or a more complicated reaction to the loss. This includes suicide ideation, severe low mood, anxiety and substance misuse. In the past these people have been denied treatment to help alleviate these symptoms because health professionals have been reluctant to label anything related to bereavement and grief as a mental illness. With growing evidence to suggest more people than first believed experience severe or intense grief reactions, and that people with a recent bereavement can still meet all the criteria of a diagnosis of major depressive disorder, the previous exclusions have been removed. In turn, it is now accepted that grief can act as a trigger to the onset of depression or that a person may be experiencing a prolonged grief disorder. This is distinct from depression in that the criteria includes a pervasive and persistent yearning for the deceased person causing impairment in daily functioning (WHO, 2019). Likewise, while the *DSM* does not define bereavement as a disorder, the diagnosis of 'persistent complex bereavement-related disorder' has been added as an appendix (American Psychiatric Association 2013). The inclusion of this new diagnosis arose from concerns by researchers and clinicians about the inappropriate association of complicated grief (as described above) with

TABLE 12.2
The differences between normal grieving process and a major
depressive episode

Grief	Major depressive episode
Waves of painful feelings that lessen in intensity and frequency over time. Often intermixed with positive memories of the deceased.	Mood and ideation are constantly negative.
Prevailing affect is one of emptiness.	A long, sustained, depressed mood and an inability to expect pleasure or happiness.
Self-esteem is usually preserved.	Feelings of worthlessness and self-loathing are common.
Suicidal ideation can occur but is generally focused on the deceased, such as a wish to join the deceased in death or feelings of guilt towards certain gaps or failures in the relationship with the deceased.	Suicidal ideation is more likely directed at self only.

Source: American Psychiatric Association 2013

anxiety, depression and post-traumatic stress disorder. For major depression to be diagnosed after a recent bereavement, the symptoms should be clearly distinguishable from the normal grieving process (see Table 12.2).

Loss for people living with mental illness

As with any illness, there are losses associated with experiencing a mental illness (e.g. loss of independence, social connection, income and wellbeing). However, with mental illness, additional losses may occur due to the stigma associated with the illness, including loss of one's sense of confidence, social standing, self-esteem and self-image. Furthermore, people with a severe and enduring mental illness may experience further losses, particularly in relation to changes in employment, independent living, social relationships and life goals.

This type of loss is what Doka (1993, 2016) refers to as *disenfranchised loss*—one that is not recognised or supported by other members of society (Doka 2016). Doka suggests that disenfranchisement occurs when a person experiences a loss but 'does not have a socially recognised right, role or capacity to grieve', resulting in the person having 'little or no opportunity to mourn publicly' (Doka 1993 p. 128). In disenfranchised loss, other people do not acknowledge the nature of, or the meaning of, the loss for the bereaved person, which inhibits the person's ability to openly grieve for their loss, or to seek and receive support from others in their mourning. Examples of losses that can be disenfranchised include miscarriage, the death of an ex-partner and adoption. For some people, grief and mourning may be affected or exacerbated by additional contributing factors. For example, losses experienced by people with mental illness may be disenfranchised or not acknowledged because of societal attitudes to mental illness; loss for Indigenous peoples may be compounded by cultural expectations and the prevalence of multiple intergenerational losses in some communities.

LOSS AND NATURAL DISASTERS

There are situations throughout life that are unexpected or change a person's view of the world. Natural disasters such as bush fires, flooding and earthquakes can result in losses of life, homes, job, a role, status and social support. These personal, social and economic losses can be overwhelming and can escalate mental health issues such as depression and anxiety. People who have lived through a natural disaster can often develop symptoms of post-traumatic stress with helplines seeing a significant increase in calls for help. There is also a link between suicide and natural disasters with the rate of suicidal behaviour increasing in the aftermath of the disaster (Horney et al 2020).

Most recently across the world, the COVID pandemic has had a significant impact on loss. Unexpected deaths, loss of freedom through restricted travel and social distancing, loss of employment, loss of relationships, and uncertainty about the future contribute to grief-related mental health issues. Not being allowed to share one's grief with others or visit friends and family at the end of life, has led to people struggling in managing their grief. Grief in such times can be undervalued and go unrecognised. People have been deprived of the rituals of mourning or spiritual practices such as attending memorials or funerals. In denying the opportunity to publicly mourn, address the loss, say 'goodbye' and gain support from others, there is an increased chance of experiencing disenfranchised grief and other grief complications (Albuquerque et al 2021).

Usual emotional resources and coping mechanisms that facilitate restoration and recovery of mental health may not be as effective during times of crisis and yet access to mental health services can become even more difficult due to the increased number of referrals. Alternative ways of meeting the needs of people and offering support are required, such as the use of technology and online psychological support. Table 12.3 offers practice recommendations related to a pandemic.

TABLE 12.3
Recommendations for practice

Change due to COVID-19	Impact	Self-disenfranchisement: Recommendations
Unexpected or sudden loss	Feelings of impotence, guilt, and shame	Validate their emotions and give space to their expression. Use memory to create compassionate feelings (e.g. recall the feelings when one has experienced the kindness of others). Help build compassionate approaches to cope with emotions (e.g. focus the attention in the present moment rather than becoming distracted by 'what ifs?') and rumination processes. Keep in mind that things and feelings change. Imagine oneself as a compassionate person speaking to a friend. Encourage the integration of the idea 'I did the best I could, with the knowledge I had'. Reach out to others and see if help is available. Understand what one can and can't control.
Depletion of emotional and coping resources	Lack of emotional safeness conditions	Offer psychoeducation on the risk factors and warning signs of common mental health disorders (e.g. anxiety and depression). Encourage people to ask for professional help. Improve access to psychological interventions, support services and social support. Promote strategies of self-care and values and meaningful future plans. Monitor the oscillation between loss-oriented coping (confronting and handling feelings of grief and loss) and restoration-oriented coping (focused on secondary stressors).

Source: Taken from Albuquerque et al 2021

LOSS ACROSS THE LIFESPAN

While children experience similar feelings of loss and grief as adults, they may express them in behaviours (e.g. bed wetting or sleep disturbances) rather than words. They need assistance in expressing their feelings and thoughts, as well as reassurance that their distress is reasonable and acceptable. Similarly, teenagers may display their distress behaviourally (e.g. mood changes, withdrawal). At the other end of the spectrum the losses experienced by elderly people can be multiple and cumulative (death of friends, loss of health/independence), which can complicate their grieving.

LOSS FOLLOWING SUICIDE

Grief following loss of a loved one to suicide can be complicated and intense due to the circumstances of the death and feelings of guilt, shame, blame and anger that can be experienced by the person's surviving family and friends. Health professionals can assist a person bereaved through suicide by offering compassion, non-judgmental support, an opportunity to tell their story (repeatedly if necessary) and recognition and validation of the person's experience of loss. Providing information about support services for survivors of suicide may also be helpful (Grieflink 2019a).

LOSS FOR INDIGENOUS PEOPLES

Losses experienced by Indigenous peoples are complex, multifaceted and frequently have intergenerational consequences. In addition to the losses that are experienced by all people, Māori and Australian Aboriginal and Torres Strait Islander peoples experience additional losses as a consequence of a history of colonisation, past trauma and separation from family, land and culture. This has led to 'unresolved or ongoing grief [being] common in Aboriginal communities because of the *unfinished business* of colonisation and the Stolen Generations' (Wynne-Jones et al 2016).

For social and historical reasons, Indigenous peoples may experience multiple losses and more-frequent death of relatives than the wider population, hence they are engaged in more frequent 'sorry business'. Furthermore, not only have Indigenous peoples suffered major losses but they have also suffered the loss of the practices and rituals that enable them to deal with those losses (GriefLink 2019b). Suggested strategies for responding to losses among Indigenous peoples are summarised in Table 12.4.

TABLE 12.4
Strategies for responding to losses among Indigenous peoples

Strategies for Indigenous peoples	How non-Indigenous people can help
Create awareness about the impact of losses and the unresolved grief on people. Create and develop grieving ceremonies suited to today. Re-create women's business/ ceremonies. Re-create men's business/ ceremonies. Re-create rites of passage (young people).	Continue to change non-Indigenous history books. Develop loss and grief counselling courses for Indigenous and non-Indigenous people. Ensure healing centres deal with Indigenous health issues from a holistic perspective. Develop loss and grief programs and workshops as a part of the curriculum within primary and secondary schools. Assist towards a true reconciliation, with the full understanding that both groups—non-Indigenous and Indigenous peoples—have deep grief. Throughout all levels of the medical profession, teach students about the complexities of Indigenous and non-Indigenous grief.

Source: GriefLink 2019b

PROFESSIONAL SUPPORT AND ASSISTING A BEREAVED PERSON

Health professionals are in the unique position of being a caregiver in the loss and bereavement experience of a person who may well be a stranger to them, and being able to facilitate the person's grieving. When providing support to a bereaved person, it is important not to interpret intense grief and mourning reactions as symptoms of mental illness. Health professionals can provide support for people experiencing uncomplicated grief by: being there for the person; allowing the person to express emotional pain; being sensitive to cultural considerations in death and dying and acknowledging the meaning of death and dying in different cultures; acknowledging difficulties; and exploring opportunities for advanced professional training. See Box 12.2 for guidelines (based on Worden's model) that health professionals can use to support a person who is grieving (Barkway & Bull 2019)

LOOKING AFTER YOURSELF

Finally, while loss and bereavement are a normal part of life for all people, health professionals are exposed to other people's losses on a regular basis, which can lead to intense emotional reactions to the distress observed (Houck 2014). Furthermore, health professionals may have experienced a loss similar to that of the person they are caring for, which can reactivate the health professional's own previous grief reaction.

Consequently, working with people experiencing loss can be stressful, and health professionals need to be mindful of managing their own mental health. This can be achieved through self-awareness, acquiring knowledge about loss and grief (e.g. regarding cultural expectations and practices) and developing helping skills (e.g. listening and acceptance) to assist the grieving person and their families. Furthermore, clinical supervision can be used to examine one's professional and personal reactions when working with a grieving person and to critically reflect on how this affects the health professional's clinical practice. And, if you experience a distressing personal response while caring for a bereaved person, there are counselling services in the workplace and the community that you can access for support.

CONCLUSION

Loss is a distressing and relatively common human experience. Though upsetting, most people's bereavement experience is uncomplicated, with only a small number of people experiencing a complicated grief reaction requiring professional intervention. The nature of the work undertaken by health professionals means you may play a role in the loss experiences of the people to whom you provide care. In such situations, health professionals can assist the bereaved by validating the loss through listening, acknowledging the person's feelings, facilitating mourning behaviours and making referrals to self-help support groups or counselling if appropriate.

REFERENCES

Albuquerque, S., Teixeira, A., & Rocha, J. (2021). COVID-19 and disenfranchised grief. *Frontiers in Psychiatry 12*, 114

American Psychiatric Association. (2013). *Diagnostic and statistical manual of mental disorders (DSM-5)*. Washington DC: American Psychiatric Publishing.

Barkway, P. & Bull M. (2019). Loss. In P. Barkway & D O'Kane (Eds.). *Psychology: an introduction for health professionals*. Sydney: Elsevier.

Doka, K. (1993). Disenfranchised grief: a mark of our time. Paper presented at the 8th Biennial Conference of the National Association for Loss and Grief (NALAG). Yeppoon, Queensland, pp. 128–132.

Doka, K. (2016). *Grief is a journey.* New York: Atria Books.

GriefLink (2019a) Grief and suicide. Online. Available: https://grieflink.org.au/factsheets/grief-and-suicide/ / 1 April 2021.

GriefLink. (2019b). Grief reactions associated with indigenous grief. Online. Available: https://grieflink.org.au/factsheets/grief-of-indigenous-people/ 1 April 2021.

Horney, J.A., Karaye, I.M, Abuabara, A., et al. (2020). The impact of natural disasters on suicide in the United States, 2003-2015. *Crisis, 0,* 1–7.

Houck, D. (2014). Helping nurses cope with grief and compassion fatigue: an educational intervention. *The Clinical Journal of Oncology Nursing, 18*(4), 454–458.

Kübler-Ross, E. (1969). *On death and dying.* London: Macmillan.

Kübler-Ross, E., & Kessler, D. (2014). *On grief and grieving.* London: Simon and Schuster.

Mead, S. M. (2016) *Tikanga Māori: living by Māori values* (revised ed.). Wellington: Huia.

Neimeyer, R. A. (2019). Meaning reconstruction in bereavement: development of a research program. *Death Studies, 43*(2), 79–91.

Worden J. W. (2018). *Grief counseling and grief therapy: a handbook for the mental health practitioner* (5th ed). New York: Springer.

World Health Organization (WHO). 2019. *International Classification of Diseases* (11th rev.) (*ICD-11*). Geneva: WHO.

Wynne-Jones, M., Hillin, A., Byers, D., et al. (2016). Aboriginal grief and loss: a review of the literature. *Australian Indigenous Health Bulletin 16*(3).

WEB RESOURCES

Australian Centre for Grief and Bereavement: www.grief.org.au. This website provides education, publications and resources about loss for health professionals and the wider community.

Centre for Loss and Grief (NALAG Australia): http://www.nalag.org.au. NALAG New Zealand: https://www.kiwifamilies.co.nz/directory/listing/national-association-for-loss-grief. NALAG is an international voluntary, non-profit organisation that focuses on issues related to loss and grief. It provides an information resource on death-related grief for the community and professionals.

Headspace: https://headspace.org.au/young-people/dealing-with-grief-and-loss-and-the-effects-on-mental-health/. This website offers information to support children and young people experiencing grief and loss.

Skylight NZ: www.skylight.org.nz. This website provides information and resources for children, families and health professionals dealing with trauma, loss and grief.

Survivors of Suicide: www.survivorsofsuicide.com. This organisation aims to help those who have lost a loved one to suicide resolve their grief and pain in their own personal way.

13 LAW AND ETHICS

INTRODUCTION

This chapter explores core legal and ethical issues concerned with the care and treatment of people with mental illness within the least restrictive environment. The intent is to provide an introduction to some of the issues rather than a comprehensive unpacking of the interplay between legal and ethical issues.

MENTAL HEALTH LAW

Mental health legislation refers to laws regarding the treatment, care and rehabilitation of people with mental illness. The legislation is designed to protect people with mental illness from inappropriate treatment and to direct the provision of mental healthcare and the services in which it is provided. Contemporary mental health legislation is underpinned by a principle that requires clinicians to use the least restrictive alternatives and to only use containment and restraint as a last resort. Most mental health legislative documents cover both the treatment and the care of voluntary and involuntary patients, and mental health is the only healthcare specialty that is governed in part by a framework of legal compulsion (Maude & O'Brien 2017). In New Zealand the legal framework is called the *Compulsory Assessment and Treatment Act 1992,* in England and Wales legislation refers to the *Mental Health Act 2007,* whereas in Australia each state and territory currently has a separate mental health Act with different requirements regarding treatment and detention. Legal regulations therefore are specific to each country or state.

Involuntary detention continues to be controversial because it involves removing a person's freedom and autonomy under the auspices of mental health legislation. Therefore, the State can compel people with mental illness to undergo treatment against their will, raising complex legal and ethical issues. The World Medical Association's *Statement on Ethical Issues Concerning Patients with Mental Illness* (2015) states that compulsory hospitalisation should only be used when it is medically necessary and for the shortest possible duration. Laws regarding involuntary hospitalisation and treatment vary worldwide; however, it is generally acknowledged that such a decision requires the following criteria to be satisfied:

1. The person is experiencing mental illness.
2. The person is a danger to self or others.
3. Immediate treatment is required.
4. Appropriate treatment in approved mental health settings is available.
5. The person has impaired decision-making capacity in relation to their mental illness.

Countries such as Australia, New Zealand, the United Kingdom and the USA use terms such as 'detained, sectioned, ordered, emergency holds, court mandated and scheduled'. These *all* refer to involuntary commitment to a psychiatric hospital for treatment, or to involuntary treatment in the community under a community treatment order. In general terms, people with mental illness can usually be committed for inpatient treatment for a short period of time; for example, seven days after examination by a qualified agent such as a medical practitioner, mental health nurse or other authorised professional. While the process can vary greatly in different countries and even different jurisdictions, most legislation requires the person to be examined again within 24 hours by a psychiatrist, who can then allow the detention to lapse or continue. With further review, the detention may be extended and, under certain circumstances, forced treatment may be instituted beyond this time, if it is felt that the person requires ongoing care and treatment in hospital or the community.

All people should receive the right to appeal their involuntary commitment or treatment order. It is common for countries to have a process where an independent decision-making body such as a tribunal board or judicial hearing can be accessed by the person being detained. These boards are often represented by a panel of mental health professionals, consumer advocates and laypeople with a primary task of ensuring a person's rights are upheld and care is delivered in the least restrictive environment. They have the power by law to decide whether a person's involuntary hospitalisation and treatment is upheld or revoked by undertaking an independent review. Similarly, they can determine whether a person's involuntary commitment is extended or that other treatment such as electroconvulsive treatment (ECT) can be delivered when a person does not have capacity for informed consent. Since everyone who is being hospitalised and treated involuntarily can appeal or apply for a review of decisions made about their detention, it is imperative for people with mental illness to be provided with information about their rights and details of advocacy groups on admission to a psychiatric inpatient facility.

These boards and tribunals also assist when a person may be unable to make decisions for themselves due to mental illness and dangerousness. In each state and territory of Australia the title and makeup are different from state to state (e.g. in New South Wales and Queensland the panel is known as the Mental Health Review Tribunal; in Victoria it is known as the Mental Health Tribunal; in South Australia it is known as the South Australian Civil and Administrative Tribunal; and in Tasmania it is known as the Guardianship and Administration Board).

In New Zealand, in accordance with the Treaty of Waitangi, section 5 of the New Zealand *Mental Health Act* requires that the cultural identity of people with mental illness is respected and attended to (Maude & O'Brien 2017). People with mental illness may *not* be involuntarily held under mental health legislation in any jurisdiction on the following grounds:

- political, religious or personal beliefs
- sexual preference
- criminal behaviour
- illegal drug use
- intellectual disability.

People with mental illness who are held against their will in a psychiatric inpatient facility must be provided with written and verbal information explaining all procedures, as well as their legal rights and how they can appeal the decision, in a language they understand. Just as other administered medical treatment requires informed consent prior to treatment, the same is applicable for those detained under a mental health Act. To give informed consent, the person must have the 'capacity' to make decisions. All people, regardless of age or legal status, are recognised as having 'capacity'. In some circumstances, however, a psychiatrist can apply a legal order to mandate a person to receive treatment as part of an involuntary admission or in the community.

There are strict criteria regarding the administration of treatment under mental health Acts if the person is deemed not to hold capacity, including the provision that the treatment provided must be the least restrictive form of treatment. Table 13.1 shows a comparison of the criteria that must be met across Australia and New Zealand before involuntary commitment and treatment can be applied.

TABLE 13.1
Involuntary commitment and treatment (ICT) criteria in Australian and New Zealand Mental Health Acts

	ACT:	NSW:	NT:	QLD:	SA:	TAS:	VIC:	WA:	NZ:
	Mental Health Act 2015 ss58, 66, 101	Mental Health Act 2007 ss12, 14, 68	Mental Health and Related Services Act 1998 s14	Mental Health Act 2016 ss3, 12	Mental Health Act 2009 s21	Mental Health Act 2013 ss6, 40	Mental Health Act 2014 s5	Mental Health Act 2014 s25	Mental Health Act (Compulsory Assessment and Treatment) Act 1992 s2: Guidelines to the MHA 2012
Mental Illness	The person has a mental illness or mental disorder, and	The person is suffering from mental illness and, owing to that illness, there are reasonable grounds for believing that care, treatment and control of the person is necessary:	The person has a mental illness and as a result of the mental illness, without the treatment the person is likely to:	The person has a mental illness; because of the person's illness, the absence of involuntary treatment, or the absence of continued involuntary treatment, is likely to result in:	The person has a mental illness and because of the mental illness, the person requires treatment for	The person has, or appears to have, a mental illness and without treatment, the mental illness will, or is likely to, seriously harm:	The person has a mental illness and because the person has mental illness the person needs immediate treatment to prevent:	The person has a mental illness for which the person is in need of treatment and because of the mental illness, there is:	Mental disorder, in relation to any person, means an abnormal state of mind (whether of a continuous or an intermittent nature), characterised by delusions, or by disorders of mood or perception or volition or cognition, of such a degree that it:

Continued

TABLE 13.1
Involuntary commitment and treatment (ICT) criteria in Australian and New Zealand Mental Health Acts—cont'd

	ACT:	NSW:	NT:	QLD:	SA:	TAS:	VIC:	WA:	NZ:
Harm	is doing, or is likely to do, serious harm to themself or someone else or	for the person's own protection from serious harm or the protection of others from serious harm and	cause serious harm to himself or herself or to someone else or	imminent serious harm to the person or others or	the person's own protection from harm (whether physical or mental and including harm involved in the continuation/deterioration of the person's condition) or to protect others from harm and	the safety of the person or others or	serious harm to the person or to another person or	a significant risk to the safety of the person or another, or a significant risk of serious harm to the person or to another or	poses a serious danger to the safety of that person or of others or
Need for care	is suffering, or is likely to suffer, serious mental or physical deterioration and	N/A	suffer serious mental or physical deterioration and	the person suffering serious mental or physical deterioration.	the person has impaired decision-making capacity relating to appropriate treatment of the person's mental illness;	the person's health and	serious deterioration in the person's mental or physical health and	a significant risk to the health of the person and	seriously diminishes the capacity of that person to take care of himself or herself or poses a serious danger to their health.

Psychiatric treatment	treatment/care/support is likely to reduce the harm or deterioration (or its likelihood) or result in an improvement in the person's condition and	N/A	the person requires treatment that is available at an approved treatment facility and	N/A	N/A	the treatment will be appropriate and effective in terms of the outcomes referred to in section 6(1) [see additional criteria] and	the immediate treatment will be provided to the person if the person is subject to a temporary treatment order or a treatment order and	treatment in the community cannot reasonably be provided to the person and	N/A
No less restrictive alternative	the treatment, care or support cannot be adequately provided in another way that would involve less restriction of the freedom of choice and movement.	no other care of a less restrictive kind, that is consistent with safe and effective care, is appropriate and reasonably available to the person.	there is no less restrictive means of ensuring that the person receives the treatment and	The main objects of the Act are to be achieved in a way that is the least restrictive of the rights and liberties of a person who has a mental illness.	there is no less restrictive means than an inpatient treatment order (ITO) of ensuring appropriate treatment of the person's illness.	the treatment cannot be adequately given except under a treatment order.	there is no less restrictive means reasonably available to enable the person to receive the immediate treatment.	the person cannot be adequately provided with treatment in a way that would involve less restriction.	Ensure that assessment and treatment occur in the least restrictive manner consistent with safety

Continued

TABLE 13.1
Involuntary commitment and treatment (ICT) criteria in Australian and New Zealand Mental Health Acts—cont'd

	ACT:	NSW:	NT:	QLD:	SA:	TAS:	VIC:	WA:	NZ:
Additional criteria	The above criteria must be satisfied before a mental health order can be made for a person with decision-making capacity (DMC) who refuses treatment, care or support; the harm or deterioration must beso seri-ous that it outweigh-sthe right to refuse. If a person lacks DMC and refuses	In consider-ing whether a person is a mentally ill person, the continuing condition of the person, including any likely dete-rioration in the person's con-dition, and the likely effect of any such de-terioration, are to be taken into account.	the per-son is not capable of giving informed consent to the treat-ment or has unrea-sonably refused to consent to the treat-ment.	The per-son does not have capacity to consent to be treated for the ill-ness.	In con-sidering whether there is no less restric-tive means than an ITO of ensuring appropriate treatment. consider-ation must be given, amongst other things, to the pros-pectsof the person receiving all neces-sary treat-ment on a voluntary basis or in compli-ance with a community treatment order.	(i) The per-son does not have DMC (ii) the treatment will pre-vent/rem-edy mental illness; or manage/ alleviate it where possible; or reduce the risks that persons with mental illness may pose to themselves or others; or monitor and evalu-ate the person's mental state.	N/A	(i) The person does not demon-strate the capacity to make a treat-ment decision about the pro-vision of the treat-ment (ii) Deci-sions re-garding ICT must be made with ref-erence to guide-lines pub-lished by the Chief Psychia-trist.	N/A

treatment, care or support, the only criteria that applies is the existence of a mental disorder or illness. Separate criteria apply to *forensic psychiatric treatment orders.*

Source: Royal Australian and New Zealand College of Psychiatrists 2017

ROLE OF PARAMEDICS, AMBULANCE OFFICERS AND POLICE OFFICERS AS AUTHORISED OFFICERS

Various professionals have a role in the care of people with mental illness as well as in providing the least restrictive means of taking a person to hospital. Paramedics, ambulance officers and the police are frequently involved in transporting people for the purposes of assessment and treatment and have particular responsibilities that include transporting people if it appears they *may* have an illness that the person has caused themselves or are at significant risk to themselves, the public, or property.

For example, in South Australia under the *Mental Health Act 2009*, authority is given to police and ambulance officers to search, restrain and use reasonable force in transporting those thought to be suffering from a mental illness for assessment and treatment. It is important to remember that health professionals, nurses, paramedics and other groups such as the police have various scopes of practice in relation to specific types of health and mental health law legislation.

Least restrictive practice

Least restrictive practice is a key factor in providing a recovery-oriented approach. Identified as best practice internationally, least restrictive practice is the minimum response required to ensure the safety of an individual or others. If restrictive practice is required, it should be for the shortest duration of time possible and as a last resort while preserving the freedom, rights and dignity of the person. Restrictive practices include physical restraint, seclusion, chemical restraint, mechanical restraint and environmental restraint (restricted access) (NDIS 2020). If the need arises for a person to be involuntarily hospitalised, this should be undertaken with the principles of least restrictive practice in mind and with any limitations placed on a person being minimal. Least restrictive practice aligns with the rights of a person to be involved and to participate as much as possible in all decisions that affect them.

The ethics of restraint

Restraint of people with mental illness is used to control and contain dangerous and disruptive behaviour. As described earlier, mental health law allows the police, paramedics and ambulance officers to restrain and use reasonable force to contain and transport people for treatment. Restraint must be exercised within a context of the least restrictive environment (to protect a person's autonomy), as well as the duty of care that must be extended by the health professional or police officer. 'Duty of care' is a legal term referring to the obligations required by people in a workplace that they adhere to a standard of reasonable care in their day-to-day work. For mental health and other health professionals this includes a need to:

- act in the best interests of others
- not act or fail to act in a way that could cause harm
- always act within your own competence and do not do something that you cannot do safely.

Therefore, if needing to physically hold or lift a person, you must have the skills and knowledge to undertake the activity. If you do not, you could be in breach of your duty of care. The use of any form of restraint—physical (physical holding), mechanical (shackles, cuffs or netting), chemical (the administration of medication to control a person's behaviour) and confinement as in seclusion—must be used as a last resort when all other options (e.g. talking, diversion) have been exhausted. Restraint should occur for the shortest possible time and there must be careful adherence to procedures. For instance, it should only be used under certain circumstances, be time-limited and can only happen in association with a reduction and elimination plan, the purpose of which is to eliminate the use of restraint for the person in care.

Compulsory community treatment

Compulsory mental health care in the community has existed for many decades in countries such as Canada, England, Australia, USA and New Zealand. It is enacted under community treatment orders (CCT). With a focus on reducing hospital readmissions, increasing engagement with services, reducing relapse and promoting recovery, these orders have the legal requirement for people with mental illness to adhere to treatment while remaining in the community. However, how effective they are for mental health and wellbeing is under ongoing scrutiny given the human rights implications and the restrictive nature when implemented. Restricting a person's liberty, requiring that the person accepts treatment, and if they do not, having the power to summon the person back into a psychiatric treatment facility are controversial issues that continue to be debated, particularly in light of evidence showing little benefit of a CCT on reducing readmission, or improving engagement with services (Barkhuizen et al 2020, Barnett et al 2018).

Summary of rights of people with mental illness

In 1991 the United Nations established principles for protecting people with mental illness. These include the right to:

- confidentiality about their personal information
- voluntary treatment wherever possible

- information about mental health Acts to be given in a verbal and written form that the person can understand
- no treatment being given without informed consent
- receive appropriate medical treatment
- the least restrictive care and restraints only being used as a last resort
- make a complaint
- specific conditions of treatment if a person is involuntarily held
- live and work in the community (adapted from OHCHR 1991).

Mental health legislation across the lifespan

Professionals tend to think only of adults when considering the legal issues of people with a mental illness and yet mental health legislation discussed in this chapter is applicable to children and young people under the age of 18, too. The involuntary commitment of young children is infrequent in comparison with adults, as the criteria required in the compulsory detainment or treatment of a person in itself occurs far less frequently than in adults. Likewise, when working with older adults, understanding the law is strongly advisable since it can bring a range of different complexities. Factors for further consideration include but are not limited to the issue of competency or capacity to consent, based on the individual's understanding of the proposed treatment and their cognitive ability to know what is involved. Consideration for age-appropriate placement, interventions and a good knowledge of law relating to parents and guardians as substitute decision makers within the jurisdiction of work practice must also be taken into account.

ETHICAL ISSUES IN MENTAL HEALTHCARE

Ethics in healthcare refers to determining the right thing to do in difficult circumstances in accordance with the standards and competencies of your health profession. All health workers are expected to be aware of the professional standards, ethical codes and competencies related to the focus of their practice (see Chapter 3). Ethical codes provide guidance to health professionals regarding their obligations to the public and the boundaries of their practice. Box 13.1 lists the main terms in ethics in mental health settings.

Exceptions to confidentiality

An exception to confidentiality is termed the 'Tarasoff rule', which is based on a famous American case that resulted in the death of a woman whose ex-boyfriend had confided to his treating psychologist that he

> **Box 13.1** Summary of the main terms in ethics in mental health settings
>
> - *Privacy.* Information provided to health professionals is safeguarded and kept private from the general public. Privacy refers to spoken and written material and all forms of healthcare records (e.g. prescriptions, x-rays, case notes).
> - *Confidentiality.* Health professionals should keep information secret about people in their care unless it needs to be shared for the purposes of giving care; in this case, personal information may be passed on.
> - *Veracity.* Health professionals should tell the truth to people in their care and not withhold or mislead in regard to giving information.
> - *Autonomy.* This refers to a person's self-determination and ability to make decisions for themselves.
> - *Informed consent.* This refers to providing information about the nature of the person's illness, the therapeutic procedures, care and treatment, including the risks, benefits and outcomes of various treatment options.
> - *Paternalism.* This refers to decisions made by medical practitioners or other health professionals that are deemed to be in the best interests of the person in the context of their illness. This is a controversial issue and a common ethical dilemma because when the principle of paternalism is applied, the principle of autonomy may be overridden.
> - *Beneficence.* Health workers should attempt to 'do good' to people in their care.
> - *Nonmaleficence.* Above all, health workers should do no harm. Health professionals have a duty of care to not cause harm to those in their care *and* to prevent or avoid harm occurring.
> - *Justice.* Care should be provided that is fair and given equally to others.

would kill her, which subsequently happened. Under the law at that time, the psychologist was not required to inform authorities or the person in potential danger. After a number of appeals to the original decision, a therapist now has a duty to protect an intended victim where information is disclosed in the context of a health setting. Thus, disclosure of confidential information in the public interest will only be justified in exceptional circumstances where the risk to one person or the public is severe. Other exceptions can include: where the patient (or his/her parent or legal guardian in the case of a person who is a minor or a mentally incompetent adult) consents to the disclosure of the information; where health professionals have knowledge of firearm injuries or possession of firearms; and where mandatory reporting of suspected child abuse is concerned.

Comparison of individual and professional views

Based on the following case study, Table 13.2 compares individual and professional views of ethical principles in mental health.

CASE STUDY

Ethical Decision Making

Jane is an 18-year-old woman who has been taken by ambulance to an emergency department in Adelaide, South Australia. Her mother called emergency services when Jane admitted taking 30 paracetamol tablets. Jane was unwilling to go to hospital, but paramedics insisted, using their rights to transfer a person to hospital for assessment if they believe a person may be suffering from a mental illness. Jane has asked ambulance staff not to tell her mother of her suicidal ideation or previous self-harming (cutting) behaviour. Jane is unwilling to stay in hospital and despite health professionals seeking her consent to stay in hospital, she refuses and is detained under the relevant mental health legislation for treatment for her mental health problems.

Comment

Confidentiality requires that the health professionals do not inform the mother about this information, as the daughter has requested. The person is an adult in a legal sense and so has autonomy regarding her decisions. Duty of care also requires that paramedics and ambulance officers inform the treating medical and mental health team of her suicidal ideation. Under mental health legislation in Australia and New Zealand, treatment can be given involuntarily for mental health issues only, not medical care per se. Medical care can be given involuntarily under duty of care and urgent necessity.

TABLE 13.2
Individual and professional views of ethical principles in mental health

Ethical principle	Jane's view	Mental health professional's view	Human rights issues
Autonomy	'I want to stay at home and decide for myself about what treatment, if any, I need.'	'Jane is extremely depressed and does not have the capacity to make decisions in her best interests.'	The right to determine one's own health decisions
Benefi-cence	'To "do good", you should help me make my own decisions and let me stay at home.'	'To "do good", we must ignore Jane's stated wishes and prevent her from harming herself.'	The right to choose between different treat-ment options
Non-maleficence	'If you admit me to hospital, you will be "doing me harm".'	'If we do not admit Jane, we will cause greater harm by allowing her physical condition to deteriorate, running the risk that she will attempt suicide.'	The right to freedom of movement
Justice	'I have the same right as anyone else to make my own de-cisions. Other people can't be forced to go to hospital if they don't want to.'	'While Jane is not able to make the best decisions for her health, we must make them for her.'	The right to refuse treatment

Source: Adapted from Happell et al 2008 p. 92

CONCLUSION

There are many competing issues for carers, people with mental illness and health professionals when caring for people with mental illness, and these are not easily resolved in many cases. This chapter has provided an overview of the central issues regarding ethics, mental health law and people with mental illness. The challenge remains to treat people with mental illness with the least restriction on their autonomy while ensuring they receive the best possible care to facilitate recovery and stability in their lives.

REFERENCES

Barkhuizen, W., Cullen, A.E., Shetty, H., et al. (2020) Community treatment orders and associations with readmission rates and duration of psychiatric hospital admission: a controlled electronic case register study. *BMJ Open*. Online. Available: https://bmjopen.bmj.com/content/bmjopen/10/3/e035121.full.pdf January 2021.

Barnett, P., Matthews, H., Lloyd-Evans, B., et al. (2018). Compulsory community treatment to reduce readmission to hospital and increase engagement with community care in people with mental illness: a systematic review and meta-analysis. *The Lancet Psychiatry, 5*(12), 1013–1022.

Happell, B., Cowin, L. S., Roper, C., et al. (2008). *Introducing mental health nursing: a consumer-oriented approach.* Sydney: Allen & Unwin.

Maude, P., & O'Brien, A. (2017). Professional, legal and ethical issues. In K. Evans, D. Nizette, & A. O'Brien (Eds.), *Psychiatric and mental health nursing* (4th ed.). Sydney: Elsevier.

NDIS Quality and Safeguards Commission. (2020). *Regulated restrictive practices guide.* Penrith, Australia: NDIS Quality and Safeguards Commission.

Office of the United Nations High Commissioner for Human Rights (OHCHR). 1991. *Principles for the protection of persons with mental illness and the improvement of mental health care.* Online. Available: www.ohchr.org/EN/ProfessionalInterest/Pages/PersonsWithMentalIllness.aspx January 2021.

Royal Australian and New Zealand College of Psychiatrists. (2017). *Involuntary commitment and treatment – mental health legislation.* Online. Available: https://www.ranzcp.org/files/resources/college_statements/mental-health-legislation-tables/1-involuntary-commitment-and-treatment-comparing-m.aspx July 2021.

World Medical Association. (2015). *Statement on ethical issues concerning patients with mental illness.* Online. Available: https://www.wma.net/policies-post/wma-statement-on-ethical-issues-concerning-patients-with-mental-illness/ January 2021.

WEB RESOURCES

Code of conduct for paramedics in Australia: https://www.paramedics.org/our-organisation/governance/code-of-conduct/.

Code of ethics for nurses in Australia: http://www.nursingmidwiferyboard.gov.au/Codes-Guidelines-Statements/Professional-standards.aspx.

Mental Health Legislation Australia and New Zealand—RANZCP: https://www.ranzcp.org/practice-education/guidelines-and-resources-for-practice/mental-health-legislation-australia-and-new-zealan

Royal College of Psychiatrists: www.rcpsych.ac.uk. This is a British website with readable, user-friendly and accurate information about mental health problems.

United Nations Convention on the rights of persons with disabilities: https://humanrights.gov.au/our-work/disability-rights/united-nations-convention-rights-persons-disabilities-uncrpd.

World Health Organization—Mental health, human rights & legislation: https://www.who.int/mental_health/policy/legislation/en/.

14 SETTINGS FOR MENTAL HEALTHCARE

INTRODUCTION

A significant proportion of mental healthcare can be self-managed or supported by informal community services such as local community centres, churches and schools. When a person experiences mental health distress that requires additional support, expertise can be accessed through formal channels such as health services specific to meet the mental health needs of people. Mental health services in developed countries have undergone major reform in recent decades. The World Health Organization (2019) has called for this reform to be worldwide. Reform has led to the *mainstreaming* of mental health services (i.e. providing mental healthcare within the general health system, not within separate psychiatric services) and a shift from the traditional biomedical treatment approach to a model in which *recovery* is the focus (Mental Health Foundation 2018).

Reform policy directs that 'people with mental health problems and mental illness will have timely access to high quality, coordinated care appropriate to their condition and circumstances, provided by the most appropriate services' (Australian Government Department of Health 2016) and the WHO (2019) recommends that 'mental health care is available at the community level for anyone who may need it'. This can include a person's home, community centres, local clinics, hospitals, or specialised services dependent on the severity and frequency of the mental health problems being experienced. Since people experiencing mental health issues or mental distress can present in all areas, the reform agenda has led to the transformation and expansion of the settings in which mental healthcare is delivered. This chapter provides an overview of some of the most common mental health settings.

MENTAL HEALTHCARE

Contemporary mental health services provide a wide range of interventions and programs including: assessment and treatment; emergency and crisis care; prevention and early intervention programs; mental health promotion initiatives; support for people and families who have ongoing mental health needs; and rehabilitation and recovery programs. Services can target specific population groups; for example, infants, children and young people, or older adults. Services that embrace a recovery framework also emphasise *mental health* and do not just focus on treating the symptoms of the person's mental illness.

Mental health services are provided in diverse settings from hospitals to schools. A broad range of health workers can include allied health professionals, social workers, support workers, general practitioners (GPs), nurses, psychiatrists and psychologists. Services and programs are delivered in both public and private hospitals, by government and non-government organisations and in both community and inpatient settings (AIHW 2017).

Stepped care

In countries such as Australia, New Zealand, UK and Wales, mental health services and the delivery of care has been designed to provide person-centred care within a model of 'stepped care'. This entails the delivery of care to match a person's current need. A person may enter a service at any step and move between the steps that most align with their recovery and least restrictive practice. Intensity and frequency of treatment, therefore, may vary accordingly. One of the core features of the stepped care model is the ability to offer a seamless continuum of care and delivery of services that meet individual needs (Marks 2021).

COMMUNITY SETTINGS

The preferred contemporary setting for providing mental healthcare is in the community whether this be a day clinic, outpatient unit, a person's home or via telehealth (Whitecross 2021). Community mental health services include primary care, mental health promotion, early intervention, acute treatment and community support services, and may be provided by public or private sector organisations.

CARE COORDINATION

The predominant model of public sector mental healthcare that is provided at the community level is care coordination. Care coordination is a way of ensuring consumer and carers receive appropriate and timely support. It is achieved by integrating and collaborating with all services involved in a person's care (Hannigan et al 2018). In the public sector, care coordination is mostly undertaken by mental health services, while in the private sector GPs and other private practitioners undertake this. Care coordination functions include:

- collaboration
- symptom management
- monitoring wellbeing and recovery
- identifying and working with risk
- collaborating with other agencies.

Generally, public sector community mental health services are structured into multidisciplinary teams that provide mental healthcare to specific population groups. While the structure of these teams and the names of the teams differ between health services, most community mental health services provide three types of intervention:

- crisis intervention
- treatment for people with acute mental illness
- ongoing care for people with enduring mental illness.

ASSESSMENT AND CRISIS INTERVENTION TEAMS

Assessment and crisis intervention services provide a single point of first contact with the mental health team and are generally available 24 hours a day, seven days a week. Referrals are accepted from any source. These services provide community-based mobile emergency response, crisis assistance, initial assessment, short-term case management, admission to psychiatric inpatient units and referral for treatment within the community.

COMMUNITY TREATMENT TEAMS

Community treatment services provide community-based multidisciplinary care coordination and consultancy services to people with mental illness and their family or carers. In addition to providing treatment for the mental illness, emphasis is placed on assisting people with mental illness to develop skills in self-care and independent living in their own environment, thereby encouraging integration within the community and recovery. They have a crisis, care coordination and rehabilitation role, which means the person is engaged with one mental health professional throughout the episode of care—that is, through the crisis and rehabilitation phases and for ongoing case management.

OUTREACH/MOBILE ASSERTIVE CARE TEAMS

Mobile assertive care services provide intensive and medium-term support to people with a severe and disabling mental illness. The services provide: intensive, mobile, community-based care coordination; specialist care regarding self-care, medication and treatment options; close liaison with other support services; linkage and advocacy with external agencies or services; and carer support and education. Outreach teams for homeless people provide mental health services for a population that might not otherwise access these services.

GENERAL PRACTITIONERS

GPs are frequently the first point of contact for people with mental health problems or mental illness. GPs can refer the person either to a private mental health practitioner or to the local public mental health service. Also, people who have been treated by public sector mental health services will often be discharged into the care of their GP for ongoing case management.

PRIVATE PRACTITIONERS

Psychiatrists, psychologists, mental health nurse practitioners and other allied health professionals in private practice provide treatment, counselling and case management services. Generally, private health insurance is required to access these services, though some private services are publicly funded.

In Australia seeing a mental health specialist such as a psychologist in private practice attracts a fee; however, if a GP develops a 'mental health treatment care plan' for the person, the fee can be subsidised via Medicare. In New Zealand private psychologists and mental health nurses deliver mental health services in primary care settings, including services such as health promotion, prevention, early intervention and treatment for mental health or addiction (New Zealand Ministry of Health 2017).

PRIMARY HEALTHCARE

Primary Health Networks (PHN) are independent organisations first established in Australia in 2015 and funded by the government. They have the responsibility for the coordination and provision of primary healthcare programs for people at risk of poor health outcomes (Happell & Platania-Phung 2019). Their overarching aim is to increase access to primary healthcare services and to help provide coordinated clinical care for people in the community who have chronic and enduring illness, including people with severe mental illness and complex needs. New Zealand similarly recognises the importance of primary healthcare with a commitment to improve access to essential services and improve population health via Primary Health Organisations (PHOs) (New Zealand Ministry of Health 2020b). Community-based practitioners who often work in primary care include occupational therapists, psychologists or credentialled mental health nurses (Australian College of Mental Health Nurses (ACMHN 2017). Such health professionals are employed to work with people with mental illness, their families and carers in a range of settings—including GP practices, private clinics, supported accommodation and private homes—to provide coordinated clinical care for people living in the community who have mental health disorders or a mental illness. They are employed within primary care to provide a range of services to enhance continuity of care, which are geared towards each person's particular needs. Services include:

- care coordination
- therapeutic interventions
- regular review of the person's mental state
- medication monitoring and management
- providing information about physical healthcare to people with mental illness and to carers
- providing education and acting as a resource regarding mental health and mental illness to other professionals within the practice (ACMHN 2017).

PHARMACISTS

Pharmacies are an easily accessible community resource. Pharmacists play a vital role to work in partnership with people with mental illness, carers and care coordinators. While recognising that medication may not be the primary or sole option for treating mental illness, the society's aim is for pharmacists to work in partnership with people with mental illness to provide direct (medication management and advice) and indirect (education and health promotion) services and, thereby, facilitate recovery (Pharmaceutical Society of Australia 2019).

NON-GOVERNMENT ORGANISATIONS

Non-government organisations (NGOs) play a significant role in providing psychosocial, support and rehabilitation services to people with mental illness, including employment, accommodation, social support, information, family respite, and day and recreation programs.

NGOs are generally run by not-for-profit organisations with the support of government funding. This sector has grown significantly in recent decades.

The support provided by NGOs assists people who are living with severe and enduring mental illness to: improve their quality of life; acquire suitable accommodation; participate to their maximum extent in social and recreational activities; pursue education and employment opportunities; and achieve an optimal level of independent living in the community. Programs also provide community access, community development and outreach support. NGOs also provide leadership and are frequently at the forefront of: innovations in service delivery; workforce culture change; effective partnerships with people with mental illness, carers, families and communities; and putting *recovery* into action (New Zealand Ministry of Health 2020a).

COMMUNITY DISABILITY SUPPORT PROGRAMS

The National Disability Insurance Scheme (NDIS) provides support for Australians aged under 65 years living with a disability (including mental illness) and their families and carers to assist the person to build the skills and capability to enable them to participate in the community and employment. Services include:

- access to mainstream and community services and supports
- assistance in maintaining informal support arrangements
- access to reasonable and necessary funded supports (NDIS 2020).

In New Zealand community support for people living with mental illness (and other disabilities) and their carers is guided by the New Zealand Disability Strategy 2016–2026 (Ministry of Social Development 2016). The core focus of the strategy is to increase choice and control in the lives of people living with disabilities and their families and to provide equal opportunities for all people in New Zealand. This latest nationwide reform employs an explicit social investment approach—that is, early monetary investment to enable better long-term life outcomes for people with mental illness, and to reduce long-term costs for government. It offers an interagency approach between health, education and social development (New Zealand Ministry of Health 2021).

MUTUAL SUPPORT/SELF-HELP/INFORMATION/ ADVOCACY GROUPS

Mutual support/self-help/information/advocacy groups offer peer-based support, information and social action services to people with mental illness and their families and carers. Skylight Australia and

Supporting Families in Mental Illness New Zealand are examples of such organisations. In addition to providing support, accommodation, employment training, friendship and psychoeducation for their members, these organisations also play a significant role in advocacy and lobbying for appropriate services for people with mental illness and challenging the stigma of mental illness as well as the consequent discrimination experienced by people with mental illness and their carers.

HOSPITAL SETTINGS

Public and private hospitals provide treatment for mental illness in specialised mental health inpatient units and in general hospital settings. People with mental illness admitted to inpatient units may be voluntary or involuntary (compelled to accept treatment under the relevant mental health Act).

Acute inpatient units

Acute inpatient units provide care for people requiring hospitalisation who cannot be supported in the community. Care is provided 24 hours a day by a multidisciplinary team of medical and allied health professionals including mental health nurses, psychiatrists, psychologists, social workers and occupational therapists.

Inpatient units are located in specialised psychiatric hospitals and within acute general hospitals. They provide individual treatment as well as a comprehensive activities program designed to meet a range of individual needs. The goals of inpatient therapy include:

- a safe environment
- structure
- support
- involvement
- validation
- symptom management
- maintaining links with the person's family or others
- developing or maintaining links with the community.

Secure/extended care inpatient facilities

Secure/extended care inpatient facilities provide a safe, supportive environment for people with serious mental illness and whose behaviours may put themselves or others at risk. The units provide intensive inpatient treatment and care to people who have persistent severe symptoms that limit their capacity to live in the community.

Intermediate care centres

Intermediate care centres, sometimes known as sub-acute residential care settings, are 'step up–step down' facilities that provide care for people living in the community who are experiencing early warning signs of a relapse, and for people leaving hospital who require a transition before returning home. The care is recovery-focused and delivered by a nurse-led multidisciplinary team in a homelike, supportive environment. The focus is on improving the person's day-to-day functioning and connection with local community services such as health, housing, employment and recreation that will support ongoing recovery and a meaningful life.

Mental health triage and consultation-liaison psychiatry

Mental health triage has both a clinical and a consultation function provided at a point of entry to a health service such as in an emergency department. It provides assessment, consultation, referral and admission if required. The service is delivered by mental health nurses, psychiatrists and allied mental health professionals who provide expert consultation and support to non-mental health professionals in hospital emergency departments or other settings.

Consultation-liaison psychiatry services are provided for people with a primary medical condition (e.g. an elderly person who develops a delirium following general anaesthesia) in general hospital settings. Services are also available for people who have a known mental illness associated with or complicated by a medical problem (e.g. a person who develops metabolic syndrome after taking an atypical antipsychotic medication). Services provided by a consultation-liaison psychiatry service include:

- mental health assessment and intervention for inpatients, including risk assessment
- advice on the acute psychiatric management of people who have attempted suicide or self-harm
- in-service education for staff on mental health issues
- advice on psychopharmacology, psychological interventions and mental health legislation (Daniel & Delgado 2021)

SPECIAL POPULATIONS

In addition to the mental health settings outlined above, mental healthcare is also delivered by specialised services that focus on the needs of particular populations and are offered across a variety of settings within both the community and institutions. These include services specifically for: infants, children and young people; elderly; prisoners; Indigenous peoples; people with specific diagnoses (e.g. eating disorders); people with drug and alcohol problems; people living in particular geographical areas (e.g. regional, remote and rural populations); and refugees and immigrants.

CONCLUSION

Contemporary health policy directs mental health service providers to deliver care for people with mental illness that is responsive to their (and their carers') needs, promotes positive outcomes and facilitates sustained recovery (Australian Government Department of Health 2016). To enable this outcome, people with mental illness and carers need access, in a timely manner, to the most appropriate clinical and community services.

Settings for delivering mental healthcare are diverse and include the community and healthcare institutions. While care in the community is advocated as the preferred setting in which to deliver mental healthcare, at times some people will require inpatient care. Finally, decisions about where to deliver care need to be made collaboratively, be person-centred and be based on the needs of the person and their family/carers to best facilitate the person's recovery.

REFERENCES

Australian College of Mental Health Nurses (ACMHN). (2017). *Credential for Practice Program.* Online. Available: http://www.acmhn.org/credentialing/what-is-credentialing April 2021.

Australian Government Department of Health. (2016). *Draft fifth national mental health plan: an agenda for collaborative government action in mental health 2017–2022.* Canberra: Commonwealth of Australia. Online. Available: http://www.health.gov.au/internet/main/publishing.nsf/content/mental-fifth-national-mental-health-plan 13 April 2021.

Australian Institute of Health and Welfare (AIHW). (2017). *Mental health services—in brief.* Cat. no. HSE 192. Canberra: AIHW.

Daniel, C., & Delgado, C. (2021). Generalist inpatient settings. In K. Foster , P. Marks, A. O'Brien & T. Raeburn (Eds.). *Psychiatric and mental health nursing* (5th ed.). Sydney: Elsevier.

Hannigan, B., Simpson, A., Coffey, M., et al. (2018). Care coordination as imagined, care coordination as done: findings from a cross-national mental health systems study. *International Journal of Integrated Care, 18*(3), 12.

Happell, B., & Platania-Phung, C. (2019). Review and analysis of the Mental Health Nurse Incentive Program. *Australian Health Review, 43*(1), 111–119.

Marks, P. (2021). Mental health in every setting. In K. Foster, P. Marks, A. O'Brien & T. Raeburn (Eds.), *Psychiatric and mental health nursing* (5th ed.). Sydney: Elsevier.

Mental Health Foundation. (2018). *Recovery.* Online. Available: https://www.mentalhealth.org.uk/a-to-z/r/recovery 13 April 2021.

Ministry of Social Development. (2016). *New Zealand Disability Strategy 2016–2026.* Online. Available: https://www.odi.govt.nz/nz-disability-strategy/about-the-strategy/new-zealand-disability-strategy-2016-2026/ 09 April 2021.

National Disability Insurance Scheme (NDIS). (2020). *Mental health.* Online. Available: https://www.ndis.gov.au/understanding/ndis-and-other-government-services/mental-health 11 April 2021.

New Zealand Ministry of Health. (2017). *Primary mental health.* Online. Available: http://www.health.govt.nz/our-work/primary-health-care/primary-health-care-subsidies-and-services/primary-mental-health 9 April 2021.

New Zealand Ministry of Health. (2020a). *Key organisations.* Online. Available: https://www.health.govt.nz/new-zealand-health-system/key-health-sector-organisations-and-people/non-governmental-organisations 11 April 2021.

New Zealand Ministry of Health. (2020b). *Primary health care.* Online. Available: https://www.health.govt.nz/our-work/primary-health-care 9 April 2020.

New Zealand Ministry of Health. (2021). *Disability services.* Online. Available: https://www.health.govt.nz/our-work/disability-services/disability-projects/disability-support-system-transformation 09 April 2021.

Pharmaceutical Society of Australia. (2019*). Response to the interim productivity commission report into mental health.* Canberra: Pharmaceutical Society of Australia Ltd.

Whitecross, F. (2021). Settings for mental health. In K. Foster, P. Marks, A. O'Brien & T. Raeburn (Eds.), *Psychiatric and mental health nursing* (5th ed.). Sydney: Elsevier.

World Health Organization (WHO). (2019). *The WHO special initiative for mental health (2019–2023): universal health coverage for mental health.* Geneva: WHO. Online. Available: https://apps.who.int/iris/handle/10665/310981 April 2021.

WEB RESOURCES

Australian Government Department of Health—Mental health: http://www.health.gov.au/internet/main/publishing.nsf/Content/Mental+Health+and+Wellbeing-1. The federal government's mental health and wellbeing homepage provides access to information about mental health reform, legislation, policy, resources, initiatives and publications.

Health boards and departments of health: See your local health board or state or territory health department website for specific details of the mental health services provided and the settings in which these services are delivered.

Headspace: https://headspace.org.au/young-people/mental-health/. This site is for young people between the ages of 12 and 25. It offers information on all aspects of mental and social health and provides resources for those in need of support.

Skylight: www.skylight.org.au. Skylight is a not-for-profit non-government organisation that provides self-help, support and advocacy for people with serious mental illnesses, their families and friends. Skylight's mission is to 'increase opportunities to achieve good mental health; to promote acceptance of mental illness in the community; and provide quality services for people with mental illness, their family and friends'.

Mental Health Foundation of New Zealand (Mauri Tu, Mauri Ora): www.mentalhealth.org.nz. This charity endeavours to foster positive mental health and wellbeing. It assists individuals, whānau, organisations and communities to improve and sustain their mental health and reach their full potential.

Mental Health Innovation Network: https://www.mhinnovation.net/community/organizations. This site offers mental health resources including a global database of organisations to improve mental health literacy and access to services.

New Zealand Ministry of Health: https://www.health.govt.nz/our-work/mental-health-and-addiction. The ministry's mental health homepage provides access to information about mental health legislation, policy, resources, publications and how to access mental healthcare.

Safewards: www.safewards.net. The Safewards model of mental healthcare originated in the UK and is being implemented worldwide. It aims to provide an inpatient environment that is safe for both clients and staff, and to reduce the use of restrictive interventions such as seclusion and restraint.

SURVIVING CLINICAL PLACEMENT

GET ORGANISED

- Research your placement before you go. Find out what you will be expected to do on your first day.
- Research how to get to the placement, travel times and parking.
- Make sure your immunisations and other physical health screening, manual handling, first aid, student ID and police clearances (aged care, children and vulnerable persons) are all completed, recorded and up to date before you begin your placement.
- Find out about the prescribed dress code (if not in uniform) and dress professionally.
- Buy at least two uniforms (new or quality second-hand) for placement.
- Invest in a good pair of shoes to increase comfort and safety, if you will be on your feet a lot.
- Read as much as you can to prepare yourself for the placement.
- Focus your learning by writing objectives for the placement.
- Use a diary on your phone, computer, iPad, notebook, etc. to record relevant information.
- During your placement, prioritise tasks on a needs basis; don't drop everything when you are asked to do something, unless it is clearly an emergency.
- Find out about commonly used abbreviations in the organisation.
- Be responsible for your own learning.

COMMUNICATION

- Arrive and leave on time.
- Ask for direction about what to do on your first day.
- Find out where you can securely place your belongings.
- Find out about security measures when finishing late at night.
- Check whether you are allowed to carry your mobile phone (turned off) or whether it will interfere with the operation of electronic equipment.

- If you are not able to attend the placement contact the organisation in advance.
- Be willing to approach people with mental illness, introduce yourself and start a conversation. People with mental health problems are no different from the rest of us.
- Be polite and respectful at all times.
- Record your supervisor/facilitator's contact details and keep them in a safe place. Contact them if they haven't contacted you in the first few days of your placement.
- Actively seek out your supervisor/facilitator and ask for feedback.
- Identify and discuss your learning goals for the placement with your supervisor/facilitator, including how these can be achieved.
- Clarify expectations about your role and what you are there to achieve.
- Don't be afraid to say 'I don't know'.
- Don't be afraid to ask questions. There is no such thing as a stupid question.
- Actively seek feedback on your work from clinicians with whom you work.
- Make the effort to get to know other members of the team.
- Get involved in your allocated team, and talk to all the people in the multidisciplinary team.
- Use your initiative! Offer your opinion. Share your knowledge of research into clinical practice.
- If you are feeling vulnerable, talk to someone about it.

PROFESSIONAL BEHAVIOUR

- Demonstrate cultural awareness and sensitivity with everyone you meet.
- Know and adhere to the rules and regulations of the placement facility.
- Be aware of the requirement of privacy and confidentiality.
- Refrain from:
  - inappropriate language and behaviour
  - being argumentative and disrespectful
  - knowingly performing procedures beyond your level of practice.
- Don't agree to keep a confidence with people for whom you are providing care.
- Don't give out personal details such as your surname, mobile telephone number or address to people for whom you are providing care.

- NEVER post material about your clinical placement in social media or online. DO NOT post photographs of yourself or people with mental illness while on placement, comments about hospitals or criticisms of other staff. Health professionals have been disciplined for inappropriate postings and you may lose your job or place in your course of study.

WORK/LIFE BALANCE AND YOUR OWN SELF-CARE

- Establish a ritual for when you come home after a shift (e.g. have a shower, change out of your uniform).
- Enjoy your time off, plan social activities, contact your friends.
- Have regular contact with your peers. This will enhance your own professional experience.
- Remember that it is normal to have setbacks; make plans to address issues.
- Don't be too hard on yourself.
- Limit your coffee and alcohol intake.
- Get lots of sleep.
- Avoid taking work home.
- Exercise regularly.
- Learn from your mistakes. You are a 'newby'! Making mistakes is okay.
- Talk to those close to you if you feel you are not coping.

WHO DOES WHAT IN MENTAL HEALTH?

ACCREDITED EXERCISE PHYSIOLOGIST

An accredited exercise physiologist works with people with mental health problems to design an exercise treatment plan to increase general fitness, reduce weight and improve mental wellbeing.

ACCREDITED PRACTISING DIETICIAN

An accredited practising dietician assesses and monitors the mental and physical health risks associated with food and nutrition. They plan and manage the nutrition and dietetic care, lifestyle and wellbeing of people with mental illness. People who have or are at risk of having metabolic comorbidities, who are overweight or who have commenced new psychotropic medication, including lithium, can be supported by this professional group in managing their nutrition.

COMMUNITY VISITOR

A community visitor is a person appointed by justice departments in Australia and New Zealand to visit inpatient and residential mental health environments. Community visitors regularly visit these facilities to promote the rights of the patients and residents, protect their interests and ensure no one is taking advantage of them.

MENTAL HEALTH NURSE

A mental health nurse has formal qualifications in mental health nursing with a focus on caring for people with mental health problems. A credentialled mental health nurse is a specialist mental health nurse with specific skills and knowledge in mental health nursing. The Credential for Practice Program is an initiative of the Australian College of Mental Health Nurses and establishes a nationally consistent recognition mechanism for specialist mental health nurses.

MENTAL HEALTH SUPPORT WORKER

A mental health support worker usually has certificate or diploma qualifications in mental health and provides mental health counselling and support to individuals, families and groups in the community. Mental health support workers provide treatment referrals for clients as well as assistance with community education, support and other activities.

MULTIDISCIPLINARY TEAMS IN MENTAL HEALTH

A multidisciplinary team comprises members from different healthcare professions with specialised skills and expertise in mental health. Members collaborate to make treatment recommendations that facilitate high-quality patient care. Multidisciplinary teams form one aspect of providing a streamlined patient journey by developing individual treatment plans that are based on 'best practice'. Multidisciplinary teams provide treatment that is focused on both the physical and the psychological needs of the person diagnosed with mental illness. These teams increasingly involve peer workers contributing to the promotion of recovery and advocacy for people with a mental health problem.

OCCUPATIONAL THERAPIST

An occupational therapist has formal qualifications in occupational therapy and works with individuals and groups to achieve the fullest potential through using purposeful activities and interventions. Occupational therapists assist people with mental illness to develop coping strategies to manage their mental health issues. In inpatient settings occupational therapists design individual and group programs and activities to enhance the person's independence in activities of daily living.

PEER CONSUMER AND CARER WORKERS

These workers have a personal, lived experience of mental illness and recovery, or care for a person living with mental illness, and are employed by public, private and community mental health organisations. Peer workers can provide information and education about mental illness, recovery and support services to people with mental illness and their families, friends and carers. Peer consumer and carer workers work in partnership with clinical staff to promote hope and recovery. Because of their life experience, such workers have expertise that professional training cannot replicate. They have job titles such as consumer or carer consultant, peer worker and peer support worker. Job specifications and titles differ in different jurisdictions, and the role of peer workers is rapidly evolving. Formal peer worker tertiary qualifications are now being offered in educational institutions.

PHARMACIST

A pharmacist assists people with mental health problems by providing support, referral and continuity of care. Pharmacists support people with mental illness regarding medication adherence and staged supply services. They conduct medication reviews and monitor side effects.

PSYCHIATRIST

A psychiatrist is a medical doctor with additional training in psychiatry. Psychiatrists specialise in the prevention, early detection and treatment of mental illness. Psychiatrists can prescribe medication, while psychologists cannot.

PSYCHOLOGIST

A psychologist has formal qualifications in psychology (the study of the mind and human behaviour) and can evaluate, diagnose and treat behaviour and mental processes. Clinical psychologists use talking therapies (e.g. cognitive behaviour therapy and psychotherapy) to alleviate symptoms of emotional distress.

PSYCHOTHERAPIST

A psychotherapist has formal qualifications in counselling and usually an additional specialisation in specific interpersonal therapies such as cognitive behaviour therapy. Psychotherapists use talking therapies to help a person improve their emotional wellbeing, to improve social skills and to overcome issues (behaviours, beliefs, compulsions or emotions) that are causing them distress. Psychotherapy is a deeper form of talking therapy than counselling and usually takes place over a longer period (months to years) than counselling (weeks to months).

PHYSIOTHERAPIST

A physiotherapist has formal qualifications in physiotherapy and has expertise in managing chronic disease, muscular skeletal conditions and acute and chronic pain common in people with mental health problems. Physiotherapists also facilitate self-management of existing conditions in order to improve mental wellbeing.

REGISTERED COUNSELLOR

A registered counsellor provides support to people with mental health problems through talking about specific problems or life difficulties.

SOCIAL WORKER

A social worker has formal qualifications in social work and works with individuals and groups who need assistance with social, economic, domestic or employment issues that may have come about due to mental illness. The aim of care is to increase mental wellbeing and quality of life.

TALKING THERAPIES

PSYCHODYNAMIC PSYCHOTHERAPY

Psychodynamic psychotherapy:

- focuses on the feelings we have about people with whom we are close (i.e. family and friends)
- involves discussing past experiences and how these may have led to our present situation
- involves new understandings, which allow the person to gain insights about how they feel and to make choices about the future.

Psychodynamic psychotherapy can be brief (one or two sessions) and focus on specific issues, or it can take place over longer periods of time (months to years in some cases).

BEHAVIOURAL PSYCHOTHERAPY

Behavioural psychotherapy focuses on changing patterns of behaviour that are bothersome to the person (e.g. avoiding certain situations such as heights, shopping centres or flying). It is often used to change behaviour in children through the use of star charts and other techniques to encourage desirable behaviours. People learn to overcome their fears by spending increasing amounts of time in the situation they fear and by learning ways of reducing their anxiety (e.g. relaxation and breathing training). Homework exercises enable new skills to be practised (e.g. breathing and keeping a diary to record feelings, thoughts and anxiety levels).

Behavioural psychotherapy is particularly effective for anxiety, panic attacks, phobias, obsessive-compulsive disorders and various kinds of social or sexual difficulties. Relief from symptoms often occurs quickly.

COGNITIVE THERAPY

Cognitive therapy focuses on changing thinking patterns. It involves close attention to the way we think about certain things, particularly focusing on thinking that affects us in a negative way and causes us to experience distressing emotions. Cognitive therapy:

- aims to replace unhelpful thoughts and feelings with more realistic and positive ones
- uses principles from behavioural learning theory and cognitive psychology

- is present- and future-oriented, and is not concerned as much with childhood or past experiences
- is thought to be very helpful with people who are depressed, are anxious or have personality disorders, and in some cases it is effective with people with schizophrenia
- is often used in combination with psychoactive medications
- is goal-oriented and time-limited, usually over a couple of months.

Cognitive therapy is mostly used in conjunction with behavioural therapy (cognitive behaviour therapy—CBT) so that thoughts and behaviour are congruent.

SOLUTION-FOCUSED THERAPY

Solution-focused therapy was originally designed for brief therapy (i.e. a few sessions). It is now also used over longer periods to help people to solve their own problems. Solution-focused therapy:

- focuses on the solution, with little emphasis on the problem
- differs from other approaches such as cognitive therapy in that it doesn't assume that a person has faulty thinking
- assumes the person is the expert, that change is inevitable and that only small changes are required.

What works for the person is a key element, as is building on a person's strengths and abilities. Talking focuses on present-oriented and future-oriented situations and experiences, using questions to develop a full understanding of the person's perspective. It has wide applications in healthcare settings, from substance abuse and depression to chronic pain.

ACCEPTANCE AND COMMITMENT THERAPY

Acceptance and commitment therapy is based on the concept of 'mindfulness', which is a mental state of full awareness that requires a focus on 'being in the moment'. This focus allows the person to calm and ground themselves. In this state the person is more able to *accept* their current situation and *commit* to an action; this assists the person to have more control and fulfilment in their life. This therapy is helpful to people with a wide range of concerns including anxiety, phobias, post-traumatic stress disorder and abuse histories.

MOTIVATIONAL INTERVIEWING

This therapy aims to overcome ambivalence that a person may have about making change in their life. It helps the person explore from their perspective the good and not so good reasons involved in making a change.

It relies on identifying the person's readiness to change and then using supportive and persuasive strategies to help the person clarify their options and actions in making changes. This therapy is helpful to people with a wide range of concerns including drug and alcohol misuse, excessive smoking and people who are ambivalent about other lifestyle changes.

DIALECTICAL BEHAVIOUR THERAPY

Originally developed to treat people with borderline personality disorders, dialectical behaviour therapy has also been found to be very effective in people who self-harm and in treating mood disorders. Dialectical behaviour therapy:

- combines aspects of cognitive behaviour therapy with mindfulness and distress tolerance
- helps people recognise various viewpoints of a situation and to reduce 'black and white' (things are either perfect or awful) thinking
- focuses on becoming aware of experiences in a more realistic way and separating experiences from worries about the past or future
- uses individual sessions and group meetings (up to two hours in length) to gain self-awareness, improve communication skills and learn how to reduce emotional distress.

FAMILY THERAPY

Family therapy is mostly used in families with children who are having problems, such as families with young offenders, and for treating gambling and eating disorders. Family therapy:

- focuses on relationships within families and within relationships
- sees the family or the couple together
- involves talking about issues in an open and honest way to develop new ways of viewing and solving problems
- usually takes place over a few months, with two therapists attending all the sessions.

NARRATIVE THERAPY/NARRATIVE PRACTICES

Narrative therapy had its origins in family therapy and is used in situations where people may have difficulty in expressing themselves. The narrative approach:

- focuses on a person's 'own story' and how this shapes their lives
- identifies a person's specific problems and how the problem has affected them (hence externalising the problem and separating it as coming from inside the person)

- encourages reflection of a person's values, hopes and potential
- through dialogue, aims to reauthor a person's experience.

The role of the counsellor is to facilitate the person examining, reflecting and changing how they perceive a problem, therefore encouraging new meanings for that person. This is an evolving modality; recent focus on the experience of 'moments' assists the person to understand their feelings and their story in an 'embodied' way, which enables the person to notice a problem and intervene (when they experience the feeling).

CREATIVE THERAPIES

Other forms of therapy include creative therapies, which involve art, crafts, music or dance. The group engages creatively and members express themselves through creative outlets.

SUPPORTING PEOPLE WITH MENTAL ILLNESS TAKING MEDICATION

Health professionals can support people with mental illness in the following ways:

- Work with the person with mental illness to identify, manage and report side effects.
- Help the person with mental illness to find a regular time to take their medication, and suggest they use their mobile phone to set a reminder.
- Write down which medicines (e.g. cough/cold medicines, anti-inflammatories) interact with their medications and explain this to the person.
- Assess each person's ability to take tablets (see Chapter 9). Suggest using a dosette or Webster pack if this is appropriate.
- Check that the person with mental illness has in-date medications and returns out-of-date medicines to the pharmacist for disposal. Out-of-date medications can be toxic.
- Encourage people with mental illness to do the following:
  - Ask their pharmacist to go through what the medication is for, when to take it and any possible side effects if they are unsure or when their medication is altered.
  - Keep a list of their medication in their purse/wallet/mobile device, and give a copy to a friend.

FURTHER READING AND RESOURCES

FURTHER READING ON MENTAL HEALTH

Frame, J. (2018). *An angel at my table: the complete autobiography.* Melbourne: Penguin.

Jenson, K. (2018). *(Don't) call me crazy: 33 voices start the conversation about mental health.* New York: Algonquin Books.

Negley, K. (2019). *Tough guys have feelings too.* Sydney: Walker Books.

Richards, K. (2013). *Madness: a memoir.* Melbourne: Penguin.

Stork, F. (2016). *The memory of light.* New York: Levine Books.

APP RESOURCES IN MENTAL HEALTH

The PsychCentral blog has a list of top 10 free mental health apps at <https://psychcentral.com/blog/top-10-free-mental-health-apps>. These are based on established interventions but they do not make claims about their impact. The apps cover such areas as anxiety, mood tracking, improving sleep and relaxation techniques.

WEB RESOURCES ON MENTAL HEALTH

Anxieties.com <www.anxieties.com>. This website provides free anxiety self-help.

ARAFMI: Mental Health Carers Australia <https://arafmi.com.au/about/>. This organisation has a network across Australian states and territories providing a diverse range of services and support to families and friends of people with mental illness. Services include respite care, support groups, counselling (telephone and in person), psychoeducation and workshops.

Australian Bipolar < http://www.bipolaraustralia.org.au/>. This is a bipolar information website.

Australian Drug Information Network (ADIN) <www.adin.com.au>. ADIN provides a central point of access to internet-based alcohol and drug information provided by prominent organisations in Australia and internationally. It is funded by the Australian Government Department of Health and Ageing as part of the *National Illicit Drug Strategy* and is managed by the Australian Drug Foundation.

Beyond Blue <www.beyondblue.org.au>. Beyond Blue is a national, independent, not-for-profit organisation working to address issues associated with depression, anxiety and related substance abuse disorders in Australia. Beyond Blue works in partnership with health services, schools, workplaces, universities, media and community organisations, as well as people living with depression, to bring together their expertise on depression.

Black Dog Institute <www.blackdoginstitute.org.au>. The institute is a not-for-profit, educational, research, clinical and community-oriented facility offering specialist expertise in depression and bipolar disorder.

Canadian Mental Health Association <https://cmha.ca/mental-health/understanding-mental-illness>. This community organisation advocates for a better understanding of mental health, offering resources to promote recovery and wellbeing.

Carers Australia <www.carersaustralia.com.au>. The purpose of Carers Australia, and the network of carers' associations in each state and territory, is to improve the lives of carers, and to provide important services such as counselling, advice, advocacy, education and training. They also promote the recognition of carers to governments, businesses and the public.

COPMI (Children of Parents with a Mental Illness) <https://www.copmi.net.au/>. This site offers resources, support and education to parents, children, young people, and family and friends to promote better mental health outcomes.

Depression Services <www.depressionservices.org.au>. Depression Services is committed 'around the clock' to improving the mental health and wellbeing of people affected by depression through providing an internet-based service offering hope and understanding, information and support.

Embrace <https://embracementalhealth.org.au/about-us>. This website provides national leadership in building greater awareness of mental health and suicide prevention among Australians from culturally and linguistically diverse backgrounds.

Headspace <www.headspace.org.au>. This website is for young people with mental health issues, as well as their families and schools.

Mental Health Foundation of New Zealand <www.mentalhealth.org.nz>. The foundation's work focuses on making mental health everybody's business. Its work is diverse and expansive, with campaigns and services that cover all aspects of mental health and wellbeing. A holistic approach is taken to mental health. The foundation provides free information and training, and is an advocate for policies and services that support people with experience of mental illness, and also their families/whānau and friends.

National Institute for Health and Care Excellence <https://www.nice.org.uk/guidance>. A national UK-based site offering guidance and advice, including best practice, in all areas of health and social care.

National Institute of Mental Health <https://www.nimh.nih.gov/health/statistics/mental-illness>. This is based in the United States and offers statistics, research and information to support a better understanding of mental health and mental illness.

Royal Australian and New Zealand College of Psychiatrists (RANZCP) <www.ranzcp.org>. RANZCP is the principal organisation representing the medical speciality of psychiatry in Australia and New Zealand. It is responsible for training, examining and awarding the Fellowship of the College qualification to medical practitioners.

SANE Australia <www.sane.org>. SANE Australia is a national charity working for a better life for people affected by mental illness.

Skylight (formerly the Mental Illness Fellowship of Australia Inc.) <www.skylight.org.au>. Skylight is a not-for-profit non-government organisation that provides self-help, support and advocacy for people with serious mental illnesses, their families and friends. Skylight's mission is to 'increase opportunities to achieve good mental health; to promote acceptance of mental illness in the community, and provide quality services for people with mental illness, their family and friends'.

Supporting Families in Mental Illness <www.supportingfamiliesnz.org.nz>. This website provides education, advocacy and support for family/whānau of people experiencing a major mental illness in New Zealand.

Victorian Mental Health Carers Network <www.carersnetwork.org.au>. The network is the peak body of organisations and individuals who support carers of people with mental health issues in Victoria. It comprises: carers or former carers linked with carer groups; representatives of statewide carer organisations with a significant carer focus; workers from carer support programs; and carer-related academics.

World Health Organization (Program and Projects; Mental Health; Disorders Management—Depression) <www.who.int/mental_health/management/depression/en/index.html>; World Health Organization (Programs and Projects; Mental Health; Disorders Management—Schizophrenia) <www.who.int/mental_health/management/schizophrenia/en/index.html>. These sites provide suggested reading about mental illness.

GLOSSARY

Anxiety: a common human experience that is a normal emotion felt in varying degrees by everyone; also a state in which people experience feelings of uneasiness, apprehension and activation of the autonomic nervous system in response to a vague, non-specific threat.

Bipolar disorder: a diagnosis outlined in *DSM-5* where a person has previously experienced at least one manic episode and a depressive episode.

Clang association: a disturbance in form of thought in which words are chosen for their sounds rather than their meanings; includes puns and rhymes.

Coexist: having more than one disorder at the same time, most commonly a mental health disorder and a substance misuse disorder. Similar terms are 'comorbid' and 'dual diagnosis'.

Comorbid: having more than one disorder at the same time, most commonly a mental health disorder and a substance misuse disorder, but can include a physical disorder, such as obesity or diabetes. Similar terms are 'coexisting disorder' and 'dual diagnosis'.

Compulsions: repetitive behaviours (e.g. handwashing, checking) or mental acts (e.g. praying, counting), the goal of which is to prevent or reduce anxiety or distress, not to provide pleasure or gratification.

Credentialled mental health nurse: a registered nurse with postgraduate mental health nursing qualifications and experience who has been awarded a 'credential' for specialist practice by the Australian or New Zealand College of Mental Health Nurses.

De-escalation: behaviour (usually learned; non-verbal or verbal) intended to reduce conflict to avoid aggression and adverse outcomes.

Delirium: a syndrome that constitutes a characteristic pattern of signs and symptoms that reduces clarity of awareness and impairs the person's ability to focus, sustain or shift attention; tends to develop quickly and fluctuates during the course of the day.

Delusion: a false, fixed belief that is inconsistent with one's social, cultural and religious beliefs and that cannot be logically reasoned with.

Depression: a disorder characterised by depressed mood, with feelings of hopelessness and helplessness, lack of pleasure or interest, appetite disturbance, sleep disturbance and fatigue.

Echolalia: a disturbance in the form of thought in which other people's words or phrases are repeated; not the same as repetition of the person's own words (perseveration).

Empathy: the capacity for understanding and appreciating the feelings, ideas and experiences of another. It involves cognition (taking the perspective of another), emotion and the physical act of observing, listening and attending.

Engagement: the process of establishing rapport with a person through interactions based on acknowledging and developing a relationship based on trust.

Fear: a response to a known threat that manifests in the same way as anxiety.

Flight of ideas: a disturbance in the form of thought in which the person's ideas are too rapid for them to express, and so their speech is usually continuous, fragmented and incoherent.

Generalised anxiety disorder (GAD): excessive anxiety and worry concerning events or activities (apprehensive expectation). This occurs more days than not for a period of at least six months, and the person finds it difficult to control.

Hallucination: a sensory perception/experience that occurs without external/environmental stimuli. Types of hallucination include visual, olfactory, tactile, auditory, somatic and gustatory.

Hypomania: a form of elevated mood that is less severe than mania.

Indigenous Australian: a person who identifies as being Aboriginal or Torres Strait Islander.

Intoxication: a reversible state that occurs when a person's intake exceeds their tolerance and produces behavioural and/or physical changes.

Major depressive disorder: a condition involving seriously depressed mood and other symptoms defined by *DSM-5* that affects all aspects of a person's bodily system and interferes significantly with their daily living activities.

Mania: a state of euphoria that results in extreme physical and mental overactivity.

Mental health: the experience of having a positive sense of self and having access to personal and social resources with which to fully engage in life and respond to life's challenges.

Mental health assessment: a comprehensive, holistic assessment based on a person's developmental, family, social, medical, recreational and employment history. It includes a mental state examination and history of current functioning and presenting problems. The person and family members or carers may contribute perspectives to this assessment. Other standardised assessments (such as specific cognitive or family assessments) may form part of a comprehensive mental health assessment.

Mental illness: an illness, diagnosed by *DSM-5* or *ICD-10* criteria, that significantly interferes with a person's cognitive, emotional or social abilities.

Negative symptoms of schizophrenia: includes signs and symptoms such as blunting of affect, avolition and anhedonia.

Neologisms: a disturbance in form of thought in which a person creates new words or expressions that have no meaning to anyone else.

Obsessions: recurrent, persistent thoughts, impulses and images that are intrusive and inappropriate and cause marked anxiety or distress in a person.

Obsessive-compulsive disorder (OCD): recurrent obsessions or compulsions that are severe enough to be time consuming or cause marked distress or significant impairment in a person.

Perseveration: a disturbance in the form of thought in which the person persistently repeats the same word or ideas; often associated with organic brain disease.

Personality: expression of feelings, thoughts and patterns of behaviour that evolve over time.

Personality traits: aspects of our personality that make us unique and interesting, differentiating us from each other.

Positive symptoms of schizophrenia: includes signs and symptoms such as delusions, hallucinations and motor disturbance.

Resilience: a person's ability to achieve good outcomes in spite of adversity, serious threats and risks.

Risk assessment or risk management: identifying and estimating risk so structured decisions can be made about how best to manage risk behaviour.

Risk factors: factors that increase vulnerability to mental illness (e.g. social inequities, stressors or discrimination).

Ruminating: having repetitive and increasingly intrusive negative thoughts and ideas that can eventually interfere with other thought processes.

Safewards: an evidence-based model of care designed to reduce conflict and containment in inpatient units.

Schizophrenia: a severe mental disorder characterised by major disturbance in thought, perception, thinking and psychosocial functioning.

Strengths: a person's resilience, aspirations, talents, abilities and uniqueness; what a person can do (and do well).

Stress: a psychological response to any demand or stressor; can be experienced as negative (distress) or positive. People can respond differently to the same stressor.

Suicide: a serious act of self-harm where the person has acted with the intention of ending their life.

Thought disorder—form, content and process: thought disorder can be assessed through the observation of speech, which can identify the amount and rate of production of thought, continuity of ideas and language production. Examples of disturbances in thought include circumstantiality, clang association, derailment (loosening of associations), echolalia, flight of ideas, neologisms, perseveration, tangentiality and thought blocking.

Trauma-informed care: a model of care that aims to avoid further traumatising consumers who have been the victims of abuse or violence.

Withdrawal: usually, but not always, associated with substance dependence. Most people going through withdrawal have a craving to readminister the substance to reduce the symptoms. It is the development of a substance-specific syndrome due to the cessation of (or reduction in) substance misuse that has been heavy and prolonged.

CREDITS

Table 2.2: Adapted from Department of Health. (2011). *Framework for recovery-oriented practice.* Melbourne: Mental Health, Drug and Alcohol Division, State Government of Victoria.

Box 2.1: CHIME framework—Recovery College Greenwich. https://www.therecoveryplace.co.uk/chime-framework/.

Table 3.1: Adapted from Department of Health. (2013). *National practice standards for the mental health workforce 2013.* Melbourne: © State Government of Victoria.

Table 4.2: Sadock, B. J., & Sadock, V. A. (2007). *Synopsis of psychiatry: behavioral sciences/clinical psychiatry* (10th ed.). Philadelphia: Lippincott, Williams and Wilkins.

Box 6.2: Morgan, S. (2013). *Risk decision-making: working with risk and implementing positive risk-taking.* Brighton: Pavilion Publishing & Media.

Box 6.3: Adapted from Hart, C. (2014). *A pocket guide to risk assessment and management.* Oxon: Routledge.

Table 8.1: Bendall, S., Phelps, A., Browne, V., et al. (2018) Trauma and young people: moving toward trauma-informed services and systems. Melbourne: Orygen, The National Centre of Excellence in Youth Mental Health.

Box 8.1: Kezelman, C. A., & Stavropoulos, P. A. (2018). *Talking about trauma: guide to conversations and screening for health and other service providers.* Sydney: Blue Knot Foundation.

Box 9.3: Elder, R., Evans, K., & Nizette, D. (Eds.). (2011). *Psychiatric and mental health nursing* (2nd ed.). Sydney: Elsevier.

Table 9.4: Usher, K. (2017). Psychopharmacology. In K. Evans., D. Nizette & A. O'Brien (Eds.), *Psychiatric and mental health nursing* (4th ed.). Sydney: Elsevier.

Box 9.4: SA Health. (2017). *Clozapine management clinical guideline.* www.sahealth.sa.gov.au/clozapine.

Box 9.8: Adapted from Baker, J. (2016). *Cochrane find no evidence for as required PRN medication for mental health inpatients.* https://www.nationalelfservice.net/treatment/medicine/cochrane-find-no-evidence-for-as-required-prn-medication-for-mental-health-inpatients.

Table 10.1: Nursing Council of New Zealand (NCNZ) / Te Kaunihera Tapuhi o Aotearoa. (2011). *Guidelines for cultural safety, the Treaty of Waitangi and Māori health in nursing education and practice* (2nd ed.). Wellington: NCNZ. http://ndhadeliver.natlib.govt.nz/delivery/DeliveryManagerServlet?dps_pid=IE6429026&dps_custom_att_1=ilsdbviewed.

Box 10.2: Adapted from Life in Mind (2021). *Culturally and linguistically diverse communities.* https://lifeinmind.org.au/about-suicide/other-population-groups/culturally-and-linguistically-diverse-communities

Boxes 10.3 and 10.4: Australian Institute of Health and Welfare. (2015). *Cultural competency in the delivery of health services for Indigenous people, Closing the Gap Clearinghouse, Issue paper no. 13.* www.aihw.gov.au/uploadedFiles/ClosingTheGap/Content/Our_publications/2015/ctgc-ip13.pdf;

Box 10.5: Australian Psychological Society. (2013). *Working with interpreters: a practice guide for psychologists.* Melbourne: APS. https://ausit.org/wp-content/uploads/2020/02/APS-Working-with-Interpreters-Practice-Guide-for-Psychologists_2013.pdf; Victorian Transcultural Mental Health (2019). *Approaching work with interpreters in mental health settings.* https://vtmh.org.au/wpcontent/uploads/2008/01/VTMHProjectreport.pdf

Figure 11.1: Firth, J., Siddiqi, N., Koyanagi, A., et al. (2019). The Lancet Psychiatry Commission: a blueprint for protecting physical health in people with mental illness. *Lancet Psychiatry, 6*(8), 675–712.

Boxes 12.1 and 12.2: Reprinted with permission from GriefLink. (2017). *Helping the bereaved.* http://www.grieflink.asn.au/helping-the-bereaved.aspx.

Box 12.2: Barkway, P. & Bull, M. (2019). Loss. In P. Barkway & D. O'Kane (Eds.), *Psychology: an introduction for health professionals.* Sydney: Elsevier, adapted from Worden, J. W. (2018). *Grief counseling and grief therapy: a handbook for the mental health practitioner* (5th ed.). New York: Springer.

Table 12.2: American Psychiatric Association. (2013). *Diagnostic and statistical manual of mental disorders (DSM-5).* Washington DC: American Psychiatric Publishing.

Table 12.3: Albuquerque, S., Teixeira, A., Rocha J. (2021). COVID-19 and disenfranchised grief. *Frontiers in Psychiatry, 12*, 114.

Table 12.4: Reprinted with permission from GriefLink. (2019). *Grief reactions associated with indigenous grief.* https://grieflink.org.au/factsheets/grief-of-indigenous-people/.

Table 13.1: Royal Australian and New Zealand College of Psychiatrists (2017). Involuntary commitment and treatment—mental health legislation. https://www.ranzcp.org/files/resources/college_statements/mental-health-legislation-tables/1-involuntary-commitment-and-treatment-comparing-m.aspx.

Table 13.2: Adapted from Happell, B., Cowin, L. S., Roper, C., et al. (2008). *Introducing mental health nursing: a consumer-oriented approach.* Sydney: Allen & Unwin.

INDEX

Page numbers followed by "*f*" indicate figures, "*t*" indicate tables, and "*b*" indicate boxes.